2 04

FINALLY
HOPEFUL

FINALLY HOPEFUL

The Personalized, Whole-Body Plan
to Find and Fix the Root Causes
of Your Depression

JAMES GREENBLATT, MD
WITH BILL GOTTLIEB, CPHC

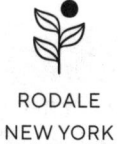

RODALE
NEW YORK

Rodale Books
An imprint of Random House
A division of Penguin Random House LLC
1745 Broadway, New York, NY 10019
rodalebooks.com | randomhousebooks.com
penguinrandomhouse.com

ISBN 978-0-593-98016-3
Ebook ISBN 978-0-593-98017-0

Printed in the United States of America

1st Printing

FIRST EDITION

BOOK TEAM: Production editor: Andy Lefkowitz • Managing editor: Allison Fox •
Production manager: Jennifer Backe • Copy editor: Dan Goff •
Proofreaders: Megha Jain, Rebecca Maines, Barbara Stussy, and Caryl Weintraub

The authorized representative in the EU for product safety and compliance
is Penguin Random House Ireland, Morrison Chambers, 32 Nassau Street,
Dublin D02 YH68, Ireland. https://eu-contact.penguin.ie

This book is dedicated to the millions of individuals and families enshrouded in the hopelessness of depression who can now find a path to sustainable recovery through Functional Psychiatry.

CONTENTS

PART THREE

MEDICAL CARE, BEHAVIORAL CARE, AND SELF-CARE

PART FOUR

A NEW APPROACH TO ANTIDEPRESSANTS

INTRODUCTION

The current medical model for the psychiatric treatment of depression is nowhere near good enough. Yes, new treatments are being researched, like faster-acting antidepressants and safer brain stimulation. But many depressed patients are still suffering. And psychiatry continues to blame patients for its own failures.

You can see this in the terminology that psychiatrists frequently use, like saying that a depressed patient has "failed treatment" or is "treatment resistant." But if a patient is taking a medication prescribed by their doctor and the patient doesn't recover—who has failed? I'd say it's the current model of care.

Psychiatry can do better. Much better. But only if clinicians and their patients take advantage of decades of largely ignored research and clinical results that show depression is not "all in your head." The research and results show that many of the root causes of depression are in your *body*. In your digestive system. In your hormone-producing endocrine system. In your immune system. And, most importantly, in your brain—and its connection to all those other systems.

Nutritional deficiencies. Hormonal deviations. Neurotransmitter imbalances. These and many other *biochemical* factors play a major role in most cases of depression.

Addressing these biochemical factors is therefore a *must* in the effective treatment of depression.

And the field of Functional Psychiatry does just that.

Functional Psychiatry bases each and every prescription and recommendation on objectively measured nutritional and metabolic factors. (Metabolism is how the body creates and uses energy.) The watchword of Functional Psychiatry: First test, then treat. And this test-and-treat approach to depression is based on *biochemical individuality*—the unique biochemistry of each person. Functional Psychiatry does not confine itself to a "one-size-fits-all" treatment, like medication. It *personalizes* treatment.

Because it is based on objective testing; because it customizes treatment to the individual; and because it employs a wide variety of therapeutic methods—

Functional Psychiatry is a uniquely powerful therapy, capable of delivering real hope and relief to people of all ages and walks of life who are suffering from depression.

Thirty Years of Treatment Success

I make this statement based on more than thirty years of experience as a Functional Psychiatrist, successfully testing and treating thousands of depressed people. During those thirty-plus years, I've learned this essential fact about depression:

> **Depression** is a *multifactorial* problem with *many* causes. Treatment often requires medication *and* therapy *and* lifestyle changes—*and* addressing biological causes, which must be detected and treated to achieve long-lasting relief.

As a Functional Psychiatrist, I don't limit myself to prescribing medications to control the symptoms of depression. I look for and detect the underlying causes of the disorder, and I address those causes using natural treatments *first* and medications *only* when necessary. And even if I do prescribe an antidepressant, I do so in conjunction with powerful natural treatments that can increase the efficacy of the medication and decrease its side effects.

In other words, as a Functional Psychiatrist, I don't take a one-size-fits-all approach to treatment—because such an approach doesn't work!

Every person with depression has a unique pattern of deficiencies and excesses that may contribute to imbalances in the brain. Correcting these deficiencies and excesses is what the Functional Psychiatry Treatment Plan is all about.

But having successfully treated thousands of people with depression using Functional Psychiatry, I'm still frustrated that there are millions of people with depression who are still searching for answers.

I wrote this book because I wanted to bring relief to as many of those people as possible.

A Treatment Manual for the Depressed Brain

Think of *Finally Hopeful* as a manual for the care and functioning of the depressed brain, teaching you how to repair the biochemical deficiencies and imbalances that can underlie depression.

I know that for a manual to *really* work in your overwhelming world—a world that presents a barrage of daily difficulties, not the least of which are the motivational challenges and fatigue of depression—the instructions have to be easy, quick, and effective. Nothing I recommend will be hard to do or take a long time. I'll walk you through a hierarchy of things to try that have been time-tested with thousands of my patients, and the thousands of patients of health professionals I've trained in Functional Psychiatry.

Part I of *Finally Hopeful*—"Psychiatry Redefined"—tells you about the disease of depression and introduces you to Functional Psychiatry. It also includes Chapter 3 (*"First Test, Then Treat"*), which provides an overview of the laboratory tests that you and your doctor can consider to uncover what is behind your depression. (Many of these tests are available direct to consumers, without a doctor.)

Part II—"Nutritional Healing"—includes seven chapters about the key nutrients I use to address nutritional deficiencies and imbalances, which are often the underlying causes of depression. All of these nutritional treatments—or what I call *targeted nutritional supplementation*—are simple and well documented. There's nothing included in this section that does not have scientific support, and that has not proven its effectiveness over decades of treating patients with depression.

Part III of *Finally Hopeful* presents the medical care, behavioral care, and self-care that you can engage in to overcome depression—from repairing the gut-brain network, to finding a therapist, to lifestyle healing with regular exercise and deep sleep.

Part IV—"A New Approach to Antidepressants"—focuses on antidepressants: how to minimize their side effects and maximize their effectiveness. It also provides a complete plan for *deprescribing*—reducing the dose of your antidepressant medication, or stopping it altogether.

If you want to end your dependence on antidepressants, you'll find the answers here.

New Treatments, New Hope

Here are some of the most important points about the Functional Psychiatry Treatment Plan that is offered in this book.

Depression is complex. Depression is a complex mental and physical condition, influenced by nutrient intake and absorption, body chemistry, metabolism, genetics, hormones, trauma, stressful life events, social support, and many other factors.

In this book, I haven't focused on the social and psychological factors that contribute to depression; they have been extensively written about elsewhere. But hardly anybody is talking about Functional Psychiatry—about the *biological* causes of depression, and how to find them and fix them. That's my focus here.

Biochemical individuality. Each person has a unique biochemistry. For example, levels of a nutrient that are considered "normal" may be too high or low for you, impeding function. For treatment to work—for depressive symptoms to clear up—the treatment has to be personalized for you.

First test, then treat. The cornerstone of Functional Psychiatry is *testing* before *treating*. Use laboratory tests to reveal the biochemical factors that underlie depression. And no factor should be overlooked—because even a slight nutritional deficiency or hormonal imbalance can trigger the symptoms of depression, or prevent full recovery. I discuss these tests throughout the book—for example, when I talk about vitamin D deficiency, I discuss the test that can detect it. And in Chapter 3, I present an overview of the most important, revealing tests. Work with this book and your health professional to determine the tests that are best for you.

Nutrition is key. Recognizing that nutrition is key to brain health is a fundamental premise of Functional Psychiatry. Identifying and correcting nutritional deficiencies often restores brain health, allowing you to live free of the symptoms of depression.

Antidepressant medications are not "magic bullets." Antidepressant medications are not a sure thing in the treatment of depression. Sometimes they work; sometimes they don't. Antidepressants are *tools* in the range of therapeutic options. At best, they are only part of the successful approach to depression. In many cases, they may not be necessary—and nondrug treatments will be sufficient.

Bottom line: Functional Psychiatry is an *integrative* approach that expands the treatment for depression to include medications *and* targeted nutritional supplementation. It also includes other treatment modalities, like therapy and lifestyle changes.

Improve the power and safety of your antidepressant. For the 40 million Americans who take an antidepressant medication, there is more good news: You can use a program of nutritional augmentation to increase the *effectiveness* of the drug, and the *safety* of the drug (helping prevent and resolve side effects). You can find this crucial information in Chapter 15. Quite honestly, it is one of my favorite chapters, because it provides so much hope and help to the many people using these medications.

You're in charge. I use words like *prescriptions* and *instructions* and *guidelines* to describe my advice. But the most accurate word is *suggestions*. I'm describing in every necessary detail what to do, but I'm not telling you what to do. You have to decide for yourself what to do. True change and lasting healing typically occur when the whole person is involved—body, intellect, feeling, and intention. Hopefully, you can appreciate how the core suggestions in this book are based on this commonsense fact: A deficiency of the nutrients required for optimal brain function will hinder healing and recovery from depression. Of course, I've been using this core principle and the resultant nutritional treatments to help patients for three decades. I hope you find principle and practice as compelling as I do.

You can partner with a health professional. You can safely and effectively implement most of the treatments in the Functional Psychiatry Treatment Plan on your own: This is a book for people who want to take charge of and clear up the symptoms of depression. But it can be very helpful to work with a health professional when managing depression, particularly when it comes to ordering and interpreting tests, and implementing protocols.

Be reassured by the science. All the treatments in the Functional Psychiatry Treatment Plan are backed by scientific evidence. In every chapter, I present a representative sampling of respected scientific studies to help give you the intellectual clarity and confidence to implement the Plan.

I also want you to know that it's not just me claiming that these methods work. It's an entire worldwide community of researchers and clinicians. These engaged experts have delved deeply into the biochemistry, neurology, and genetics of depression—and they've understood the obvious but overlooked role of nutrients and other biochemical factors in the well-being of body and brain. They've studied thousands of patients with depression to objectively test their findings and theories. And they've inspired me to synthesize their effective results—results I've been implementing in my own practice for more than three decades—into the practical advice offered in *Finally Hopeful*.

To help give *your* doctor confidence in the Functional Psychiatry Treatment Plan, each chapter provides plenty of scientific support for the treatments. If you or your doctor want to take a closer look at any of the studies I've summarized, please see the Notes at the back of the book for the study citations. You can find those same citations on my website, www.jamesgreenblattmd.com.

Prevention is possible. If you have a family history of depression but you're not currently depressed, don't wait until depression develops. Find out if you have biochemical factors that predispose you to depression. And work with your doctor to correct them.

Enjoy the results. With the Functional Psychiatry Treatment Plan, you'll experience significant results.

Your feelings of sadness and hopelessness, of irritation and discouragement, will start to dissipate, and your mood will brighten.

Your fatigue will ease, and you'll feel more energetic.

Your motivation will return, along with your ability to take pleasure in daily activities.

Your concentration and decision-making will improve.

You won't find yourself feeling worthless or guilty.

And much more.

I wish you well in this journey to happiness. As of now, we're on this journey together.

PART ONE

PSYCHIATRY REDEFINED

CHAPTER 1

Understanding Depression

> The first essential step in healing your depression is knowing the *real* causes.

This book is about overcoming depression and feeling good again. You'll learn how to create a *personalized* Functional Psychiatry Treatment Plan—an *individualized* plan of self-care and professional care. A plan that will address the unique, underlying, root causes of *your* depression. A plan that is much more than just trying to manage symptoms with a one-size-fits-all medication.

This chapter is about *understanding* depression as it is clinically diagnosed—the many types, and their many causes, including biochemical imbalances. Understanding your condition and what *really* causes it is one of the first steps in overcoming depression.

My patient Laura is a good example of what happens when you *really* understand the causes of *your* depression—and a good example of the effectiveness of the Functional Psychiatry Treatment Plan in addressing those causes.

Depressed, Bingeing, and Fatigued

Laura was a forty-one-year-old with a history of depression. She'd always struggled with binge eating, but after she was prescribed the antidepressant Paxil (paroxetine), she felt like she was in less control over resisting certain foods (particularly carbs). She had gained fifty-five pounds in the past three years. (Weight gain is a common side effect of the class of antidepressants called SSRIs, or selective serotonin reuptake inhibitors, affecting an estimated 25 percent of patients who take these drugs.) Her doctor added Wellbutrin (bupropion), an antidepressant that can help manage weight gain problems. But Laura still continued to struggle with episodes of bingeing—and continued to gain weight.

Because Paxil was making Laura's problems worse, she had been trying to wean herself off the antidepressant medication with the help of her doctor. But the effects of tapering her medication were severe, as they often are. She and her doctor had reduced the dose of Paxil from 30 milligrams (mg) to 10 mg a day. But even at 10 mg Laura was experiencing side effects—insomnia, increased anxiety, and occasional brain sensations much like electric shocks. At that point, she decided to see me.

I listened as Laura described her concerns: her depression, her binge eating, and the side effects from deprescribing. (You can read more about deprescribing side effects—and how to stop them—in Chapters 16 and 17.) I explained to her my approach—*first test, then treat*—and we discussed a range of laboratory tests that I thought would be relevant to her situation. Laura requested them all.

Revealing Results

The laboratory testing revealed several biological imbalances that were probably contributing to both her depression and her binge eating.

Vitamin B12. Laura had a very low level of B12, which in turn boosted her levels of homocysteine, a metabolic byproduct of the breakdown of the amino acid cysteine. High levels of homocysteine are neurotoxic—and high levels are commonly found in people with (you guessed it) depression and binge eating.

Vitamin D. Laura also had a very low level of vitamin D, a precursor to serotonin, a neurotransmitter that plays a key role in mood, appetite, and sleep.

Food sensitivity. Laura had a food sensitivity to eggs, which she ate daily. Food sensitivities can disrupt the brain's biochemical balance, impacting mood and potentially contributing to depression.

Kryptopyrroles. She had high levels of this chemical, a condition called pyroluria. Kryptopyrroles can bind with vitamin B6 and zinc, forcing those key, brain-nourishing nutrients out of the body. In my clinical experience, patients with pyroluria struggle with more intense symptoms during antidepressant deprescribing.

The Functional Psychiatry Treatment Plan

At her second office visit, a few weeks later, I prescribed for Laura her individualized Functional Psychiatry Treatment Plan, based on her lab results. It included:

Curcumin. I prescribed 300 mg of curcumin, two times per day, using the supplement CurcumaSorb Mind, from Pure Encapsulations, which delivers both curcumin and other therapeutic plant compounds. Curcumin is the active ingredient in the spice turmeric, and it can help control kryptopyrroles. Research also shows it can improve mood and help balance appetite in patients with binge eating.

Zinc and B6. To counter the nutrient-stealing effects of kryptopyrroles, I also prescribed zinc (30 mg daily) and vitamin B6 (50 mg, twice daily).

B12. To counter her low levels of vitamin B12 and high levels of homocysteine, I prescribed a highly absorbable, sublingual form of vitamin B12: Pure Melt B12 Folate from Pure Encapsulations. It also contains L-methylfolate (a form of folate that isn't affected by a common genetic mutation that stops the absorption of folic acid), which helps drive down homocysteine.

Vitamin D. To boost her low levels of vitamin D, I prescribed 5,000 IU daily of the nutrient.

Magnesium glycinate. This mineral supports vitamin D in producing serotonin, and is known to help with depression.

Eliminating eggs. This dietary change was intended to help stabilize her brain chemistry.

Laura readily agreed to implement this protocol.

Two months later: Remarkable improvement

I saw Laura two months later—and her improvement was remarkable. Her mood was more upbeat. Her anxiety had decreased. But most importantly to her, the episodes of bingeing were mostly under control, and she had started to lose weight. Plus, the side effects from Paxil deprescribing had stopped, and she was ready to lower the dose even further, which we did, getting her off Paxil over the next few months.

Without the Functional Psychiatry Treatment Plan—without *first* testing, and *then* treating—it's likely Laura would still be struggling with depression, binge eating, and the side effects of deprescribing. With her personalized Functional Psychiatry Treatment Plan, she was well on the way to recovery.

The same type of success can happen for you—and for any of the seventy million Americans who will experience depression during their lifetime. But what happened for Laura is not typically what happens when a person visits a traditional psychiatrist.

The Limitations of Traditional Psychiatry

What happens when a patient with depression visits a traditional psychiatrist?

Imagine that patient is you, and you are stepping into the psychiatrist's office. For whatever reason—because you feel depressed; because a family member has noticed how depressed you are and urged you to see a psychiatrist; because your primary care physician has referred you—you've made the decision to seek medical treatment.

One of the first things you notice when you enter the psychiatrist's office is that it's not like most medical offices. There is no stethoscope hanging from a hook, or a blood pressure cuff on a side table, or other instruments that doctors typically use to take measurements of patients. Instead, there is the psychiatrist behind their desk, you in a chair in front of the desk—and a box of tissues on the desk. Clearly, this is not going to be a standard medical exam, despite the fact that psychiatrists are medical doctors who go to four years of medical school, followed by at least four years of special training in psychiatry.

The doctor sits down, offers you a seat, and encourages you to describe your symptoms, and then interviews you to get the additional information needed to make a diagnosis.

Maybe you start to wonder, "What *is* a psychiatric diagnosis?" Maybe you wonder how a psychiatrist can even make a diagnosis based only on a conversation, rather than from a physical exam or test results. But that's the way it's always been done, so you go along with the program.

After your session, the psychiatrist may consult the DSM-5-TR, the big blue book that sits behind them on a bookshelf. The doctor is seeking to match the symptoms you described with one of the lists of symptoms in the book in order to arrive at an official diagnosis and to formulate an approach to your treatment.

What *didn't* happen at this office visit?

The traditional psychiatrist probably didn't ask you about your medical illnesses and physical symptoms, or those of your family. They didn't give you a physical exam. They didn't ask what you typically eat. They didn't do any lab work to check your nutritional status or hormone levels. They didn't ask what chemicals you might be exposed to at work or home, or measure toxins that may have built up in your body.

In short, the traditional psychiatrist operated on the principle that the brain is the brain and the body is the body—and neither has much to do with the other. According to this traditional view, your problem is *emotional.* Your problem is *behavioral.* Your problem is not physical. And this separation of brain and body often prevents traditional psychiatrists from finding the *real cause* of depression, or treating it effectively.

In fact, traditional psychiatrists often make treatment decisions for depression based on guesses, prescribing one medicine after another, hoping that one medication, or some combination of medications, will work. Many depressed patients take multiple psychiatric medications over time and may even be prescribed two or more antidepressants simultaneously—in addition to medications for sleep and anxiety. Research shows that nearly 60 percent of visits to psychiatrists result in two or more prescriptions for psychiatric medications. About one-third of visits result in three or more prescriptions. And if those prescriptions don't solve the problem, new medications are offered. This approach—called *polypharmacy*—is the sad reality of traditional treatment for depression.

Now, I am not against medication. The problem is not the medications themselves. It's the way in which they are used. Antidepressants can help restore health when they are used as *part* of an overall treatment plan that uses every tool at a doctor's and patient's disposal. But as with Laura, a rational, effective treatment plan is based on discovering the *real causes* of a patient's depression. Nothing else is likely to work long-term.

What are those causes?

Understanding Depression

What is the cause of depression?

Well, there are *many* possible answers to that question.

There are *psychological causes*, like childhood trauma, persistent negative thinking, and low self-esteem.

There are *social causes*, like rocky relationships and losing your job.

There are *lifestyle causes*, like poor sleep and lack of exercise.

There are *medical causes*, like diabetes, heart disease, and drug side effects.

And then there are the causes I emphasize in my medical practice and in this book—*biological causes*, like nutritional deficiencies, chronic infections, and genetic mutations (to name just a few).

Biological causes are far more common—and far more important—than most doctors think. In fact, aside from lower levels of the neurotransmitter serotonin—a biological cause addressed by antidepressant medication—most doctors aren't even aware that depression *has* biological causes.

That's because, as I've just explained, the conventional diagnosis of depression typically focuses on *subjective factors*—the patient's self-reported symptoms. And conventional medicine then provides symptomatic relief with medications. The biological causes of depression—the objective factors—are never explored.

But as you use *Finally Hopeful* and the Functional Psychiatry Treatment Plan to feel better, it's important to know not only the causes of depression, but also more about your disorder. What is depression, exactly?

Depression isn't just feeling sad. Depression is a medical disorder, and a serious one at that. In America, depression is the *leading* cause of disability from adolescence through middle age.

An estimated twenty-one million American adults experience a major depressive episode each year.[1]

Seventy million Americans will experience major depression at some point in their lives—one in four women, and one in ten men.[2]

Tragically, an estimated 15 percent of those individuals will complete suicide.[3] Suicide is the eleventh leading cause of death in America,[4] taking some fifty thousand lives every year.[5]

Antidepressants are the go-to treatment for depression. Thirty-three million Americans take them, about one in eight of us.[6] They are *the* most commonly prescribed drug among Americans between the ages of twenty and fifty-nine, and the third most commonly prescribed drug overall.[7]

But this common, destructive condition remains *under*diagnosed and *under*treated.

Millions of depressed people never see a mental health professional.

Forty to 70 percent of patients who see a mental health professional and get a prescription for antidepressants *don't* respond to the drug, or respond only partially.[8]

About half of patients who achieve full remission from major depression relapse within two years—despite being on antidepressants.[9]

The Many Causes of Depression

As I've said several times (and will continue saying throughout the book, because it's so important to your recovery), depression is rarely due to a single cause. Rather, it's usually caused by a *combination* of factors—biochemical, psychological, genetic, and many more. Let's take a closer look.

Imbalanced neurotransmitters

Brain scans show that the brains of people with depression function differently than those without the disorder, particularly in the areas of the brain that regulate mood, behavior, appetite, sleep, and thinking. The likely cause: imbalances in levels of brain chemicals called *neurotransmitters*—specifically, serotonin, norepinephrine, and dopamine. These chemicals relay messages from one neuron to the next. When levels of neurotransmitters are imbalanced, the brain functions suboptimally, like a car stuck in first gear. The symptoms of depression—from low mood to lack of motivation to fatigue—are the result. It is this imbalance in neurotransmitters that is the main focus of this book.

Many factors can cause imbalances in neurotransmitters. They include:

- chronic stress, a problem we're all too familiar with;

- poor diet, like too little protein;

- nutritional deficiencies, like low blood levels of vitamin D;

- genetic mutations;

- medications, alcohol, and recreational drugs;

- too little sleep;

- chronic low-grade inflammation, causing neuroinflammation;

- neurodegenerative diseases, like Parkinson's and Alzheimer's;

- environmental toxins;

- an imbalance of gut bacteria (dysbiosis), weakening the gut-brain axis;

- chronic illness, like diabetes or autoimmune diseases; and

- aging.

Because so many factors can cause biology-based brain imbalances, the mantra of the Functional Psychiatry Treatment Plan is *first test, then treat*. It's crucial to have a range of tests to help you *find* the underlying biochemical causes of depression—so each cause can be *fixed*. That's what worked for Laura, and it can work for you.

Medical conditions

Many different diseases can cause or complicate depression. For example, up to 30 percent of people with cancer; 45 percent of those with heart disease; 60 percent of people who have had a stroke; and 30 percent of those with chronic pain are likely to be depressed.[10] If you have a chronic disease *and* you're depressed, it's important to address both problems.

Medications

Depression can be a side effect of many medications, including corticosteroids, chemotherapeutic drugs for cancer, and even some psychiatric medications. If you're depressed, ask your primary care physician if there are any medications you're taking that might be causing or contributing to the problem.

Hormonal imbalances

The hormone-generating endocrine system sends messages throughout the body, regulating every function. Even a slight imbalance—low levels of thyroid hormones; imbalances of estrogen and progesterone; low testosterone—can trigger depression.

Genetic factors

In many cases, depression is an *inherited disease*. It's estimated that 40 to 50 percent of the risk for major depressive disorder (MDD) is inherited, particularly for severe depression.

Genetic mutations contribute to depression in many ways. A mutation can reduce the activity of neurotransmitters like serotonin; cut levels of brain-derived neurotrophic factor, which helps brain cells grow and thrive; disturb the circadian rhythms that regulate the sleep/wake cycle; block the absorption of folate, a B vitamin critical to maintaining positive mood; and more.

There are also *epigenetic* influences: There are no mutations, but environmental factors like toxins activate genes that negatively affect mood and weaken the response to stress.

Psychological and social factors

Our lives are complex, and for some people psychological and social factors—from loneliness to low self-esteem—can increase the risk and severity of depression.

Diagnosing Depression

Depression isn't one disorder. There are many different types of depression, as defined by the Diagnostic and Statistical Manual of Mental Disorders (DSM), which psychiatrists use to make psychiatric diagnoses. The current edition, DSM-5-TR (Text Revision), was published in 2022.

Let's review some of the most common types of depression found in the DSM-5-TR.

Major depressive disorder (MDD)

The diagnostic criteria for MDD include the following symptoms:

- Feeling sad, empty, hopeless, irritable, or discouraged

- Noticeably reduced interest or pleasure in almost all activities once enjoyed

- Significant unintended weight change

- Difficulty sleeping or sleeping excessively

- Agitation/restlessness or slowed movements and speech

- Fatigue or loss of energy

- Feeling worthless or excessively guilty

- Difficulty thinking, concentrating, or making decisions

- Frequent thoughts of death

To make a diagnosis, these symptoms must be present for most of the day, nearly every day, for at least two consecutive weeks. At least one of the first two symptoms on the above list, and at least five other symptoms, must be present. A diagnosis based on a single episode is possible, although most people have several episodes.

Every year in the United States, an estimated twenty-one million adults and 4.1 million adolescents have at least one episode of MDD.

Persistent depressive disorder (PDD)

The main characteristic of PDD (formerly called *dysthymia*) is depressed mood for most of the day, for more days than not, for at least two years.

In children and adolescents, mood can be irritable, and the duration must be at least one year.

Episodes of major depression may occur *before* PDD, and major depressive episodes may occur *during* PDD; when these two disorders occur together, it's called *double depression.*

About 2 percent of Americans—seven million people—suffer from PDD.[11]

Depression with seasonal pattern (seasonal affective disorder, or SAD)

SAD is present when there is a link between the start of depressive episodes and a particular time of year, usually the winter. Symptoms of MDD that occur in a seasonal pattern include not only feelings of sadness and hopelessness, but also loss of energy, sleeping too much, overeating, weight gain, and a craving for carbohydrates.

It's likely that reduced daylight and sunlight exposure during the winter trigger underlying biological processes that in turn cause SAD. In America, SAD is more common in people living in northern latitudes— like Chicago or New York City—where light is particularly reduced during the winter months.

The Three Faces of Major Depression

Mild, Moderate, and Severe

There are three types of major depression as defined by the DSM-5-TR: mild, moderate, and severe. A clinician determines the type using two basic criteria: the number of symptoms; and the degree to which the symptoms interfere with daily functioning, like work and relationships.

Mild. There are few symptoms beyond the minimum required for diagnosis, and the symptoms are distressing but manageable, with minimal impairment in daily life. *Example:* You feel sadness and fatigue, but you can still perform daily activities.

Moderate. There may be more symptoms, or their severity may be greater. Functional impairment is noticeable but not debilitating. *Example:* You struggle with work and relationships because your energy is low and you're having difficulty concentrating.

Severe. You have multiple symptoms, and they're intense and debilitating, with major impairment in functioning. *Example:* You're unable to get out of bed or interact socially.

These criteria are useful for two reasons: If you realize you have mild or moderate major depression, you can use the Functional Psychiatry Treatment Plan to treat the problem *before* it becomes severe. If you have severe depression, it's likely you'll need the targeted nutritional supplementation of Functional Psychiatry, medication, and therapy to help you move forward to a more positive life.

SAD may begin at any age, but the average age of onset is eighteen to thirty.

Approximately thirteen million Americans experience SAD every year.[12]

Depressive disorder with peripartum onset (postpartum depression, or PD)

For many women, having a baby is emotionally stressful, with up to 70 percent of all new mothers experiencing the "baby blues." This condition is short-term, lasting a few days to two weeks after birth, with symptoms of worry, unhappiness, and fatigue.

At first, a woman with PD may seem to have the baby blues—but with PD, symptoms become worse and last longer. Women with PD may have the following symptoms during pregnancy or in the four weeks following pregnancy:

- Sluggishness and fatigue

- Feeling sad, hopeless, helpless, or worthless

- Anxiety

- Difficulty sleeping/sleeping too much

- Changes in appetite

- Difficulty concentrating/confusion

- Crying for no reason

- Lack of interest in the baby or in family and friends

- Fear of harming the baby or oneself

- Difficulty bonding with the baby

There are many possible causes and contributing factors in PD, including the rapid changes in hormone levels after delivery, a lack of sleep, an insufficient support system, low blood levels of omega-3 fatty acids, and a family history of depression.

An estimated 10 to 20 percent of new mothers experience PD.[13]

Premenstrual dysphoric disorder (PDD)

Many women experience emotional and physical changes around the time of their period. For some women, these changes disrupt their lives—and can even be disabling.

To make the diagnosis of PDD, symptoms must be present in most menstrual cycles and in the week before the period, and they must start to improve a few days after the period begins and become minimal or absent in the week after. One or more of the following symptoms must be present:

- Emotional changes (mood swings, feeling suddenly sad or tearful, or increased sensitivity to rejection)

- Irritability, anger, or increased conflicts with others

- Depressed mood, feelings of hopelessness, or self-deprecating thoughts

- Anxiety, tension, or feeling on edge

One or more of the following symptoms must also be present, and they must total at least five symptoms when combined with the symptoms listed above:

- Decreased interest in usual activities

- Difficulty concentrating

- Lack of energy

- Change in appetite, overeating, or specific food cravings

- Difficulty sleeping or sleeping too much

- Feeling overwhelmed or out of control

- Physical symptoms such as breast tenderness or swelling, joint or muscle pain, or bloating or weight gain

These symptoms are linked to significant distress or interfere with work, school, usual social activities, or relationships. Many women report the symptoms worsen as they approach menopause.

About 3 to 8 percent of menstruating women in the United States have PDD.[14]

There are many more types of depressive disorders, like substance/medication-induced depression, psychotic depression, and atypical depression. (Bipolar disorder, which typically includes depression, is in its own category, and is not included with depressive disorders in the DSM-5-TR.) But the types I just described are among the most common.

But whatever the type of depression, or the cause, the Functional Psychiatry Treatment Plan can help provide relief—because this plan is customized and personalized to address the causes that underlie *your* depression, rather than applying a one-size-fits-all solution. Now is the time for true healing to begin.

CHAPTER 2

Psychiatry Redefined

The Future of Mental Healing Is Now

> *Functional medicine*—which combines medical science with nutritional and metabolic therapies—is the key to ending the epidemic of depression.

The ideas and practical information in this book offer the possibility of *real and sustained relief* from depression—a way forward to a happier, healthier life.

Now, I'm guessing you might feel a little bit (or very) skeptical about such a statement.

If you're anything like my depressed patients, you've probably allowed yourself to feel hopeful about the promise of relief from the newest drug or therapy. And then you've experienced the *reality* of the new treatment—and it's been very disappointing. In fact, research shows that up to two-thirds of people with depression *do not* respond to their first antidepressant prescription. And it doesn't get much better from there. An estimated 30 percent don't respond to their second antidepressant. Or their third. Or their fourth.[1] Conventional medicine calls these patients "treatment resistant." As I said earlier, that's a term I really (really) dislike, because it blames the patient for their "resistance" to treatment. It's the failure of the medication, not the person taking the medication!

Well, I want you to know that I understand your dilemma—because for more than thirty years, I've been successfully treating depressed patients who came to me because they didn't find relief with conventional medicine.

Young children who told me they would rather die than live with being "so sad." Teens who cut themselves to feel anything other than their depression. Adults who could no longer function at work, or whose relationships had been destroyed by the bleak atmosphere of depression. Depressed seniors, who felt like their lives were fading away.

People for whom traditional treatment had failed, and who were seeking another, different way. People who saw their depression lift and their hope in life be restored—because I treated them with a new, effective protocol called *Functional Psychiatry*.

What Is Functional Psychiatry?

I am one of the champions of Functional Psychiatry. (In fact, I was the first psychiatrist to use the term.) I have trained thousands of other clinicians in Functional Psychiatry, through my educational platform, Psychiatry Redefined. So, what is Functional Psychiatry, exactly?

It is *not* a particular drug or therapy.

It is *not* a single treatment for the complex illness of depression.

Functional Psychiatry recognizes that depression has *many* causes, often requiring a range of therapies, including medications if needed.

Functional Psychiatry understands that biochemical deficiencies and imbalances deeply affect the brain, and are among the many underlying causes of depression. Those deficiencies and imbalances also hinder recovery with medications and therapy. What are these deficiencies and imbalances?

Nutritional deficiencies. Hormonal imbalances. Chronic inflammation. Gut problems. Poor sleep. Food allergies. Chronic, undetected infections. Genetic mutations. Sedentary living. Toxins. And many more.

To identify and address *all* these factors, the credo of Functional Psychiatry is: *First test, then treat.*

Test, to *find* the deficiencies and imbalances.

What's in a Name?

Functional Psychiatry is only one of many terms for an approach to mental health that does not use a "one-size-fits-all" approach (like a medication), but emphasizes discovering and treating the underlying, root causes of mental disorders and illness. Here are some of the other names you might see being used to describe this type of approach. In a sense, these names describe *subsets* of Functional Psychiatry, which utilizes all of the following approaches:

Integrative psychiatry. This is the use of research-supported, non-pharmaceutical treatments for mental health that are *integrated* or combined with conventional pharmaceuticals and psychotherapy. Common examples of integrative psychiatry include the therapeutic use of mindfulness-based stress reduction (MBSR), yoga, and lifestyle changes like regular exercise.

A study published in the January 23, 2024, issue of *BMC Public Health* looked at sixty elderly people with depression, dividing them into two groups. One group attended weekly sessions of MBSR, and the other didn't. After eight weeks, there was a "significant reduction in depressive symptoms," wrote the researchers. The people practicing MBSR also improved in "emotional regulation" (less anger, more acceptance, and better problem-solving) and slept better.[2]

Metabolic psychiatry. This approach focuses on treating mental illness by improving *metabolism*—how the body uses (or fails to use) energy. For example, a metabolic psychiatrist might treat depression by balancing blood sugar and reducing chronic inflammation through a ketogenic diet and lifestyle recommendations.

Case history: A sixty-five-year-old woman had been struggling with depression and type 2 diabetes for twenty-six years. She was on both a diabetes medication and an antidepressant—but she still had uncontrolled diabetes, and she still struggled with depressive symptoms. Her metabolic psychiatrist recommended a ketogenic diet, an exercise program, and therapeutic counseling. Within three months of making these changes, the woman no longer qualified for a diagnosis of either diabetes or depression—her blood sugar levels had normalized, and testing showed that her depression score had dropped from 17 to zero. This case study appeared in the journal *Diabetes & Metabolic Syndrome: Clinical Research & Reviews*.[3]

Nutritional psychiatry. This approach identifies and treats common nutritional deficiencies that cause or contribute to depressive symptoms. For example, deficiencies in vitamin D, vitamin B12, folate, magnesium, zinc, iron, and other nutrients can contribute to mental health symptoms—and are often overlooked. With proper testing and treatment, these issues can be identified and treated, improving or resolving a patient's mental health concerns.

Recent study: In a study in *Magnesium Research*, a combination of magnesium and vitamin D supplementation reduced depressive symptoms in middle-aged people with long-COVID by 69 percent, compared to a 29 percent reduction in a control group not receiving the nutrients.[4]

Treat, to *fix* them.

Which leads us to another credo of Functional Psychiatry: biochemical individuality.

Biochemical individuality

This core concept behind Functional Psychiatry was originally championed by biochemist Robert Williams, PhD, in his groundbreaking book *You Are Extraordinary*, first published in 1956, and republished in 1998 under the name *Biochemical Individuality: The Key to Understanding What Shapes Your Health*.

This book has been an inspiration for me throughout my career—a revelatory source of scientific truth; and a call to practice a new and different kind of medicine that takes into account a central fact of health and healing that is largely overlooked by the "one-size-fits-all" philosophy of conventional medicine.

I'll never forget reading through the book and arriving at a page of startling black-and-white drawings. The drawings featured "A 'Textbook' Stomach," with the classic J-curve, and twelve other stomachs that looked nothing like a stomach "should" look—but were the actual shapes of people's stomachs! Dr. Williams wrote, "Here are pictures of twelve real stomachs in contrast to the 'textbook' stomach at the top of the page. These real stomachs neither look alike nor do they operate alike."

What does biochemical individuality tell us?

Contrary to what conventional psychiatry affirms, there is no "textbook" depression—and no "textbook" way to treat it.

Rather, there are (in Williams's words) "real individuals" whose bodies and brains don't "look alike" or "operate alike."

Which means that any truly effective treatment for depression has to take biochemical individuality—the real person—fully into account.

This type of individualized medicine, which is becoming increasingly recognized in all fields of health, is also called "personalized medicine" or "precision medicine."

Functional Psychiatry is the psychiatric form of personalized, precision medicine.

By first testing the individual to discover their *unique* combination of factors that trigger depression, we can provide much more than symptom relief. Rather, we treat the *root causes* of depression—which, in many cases, puts the disease into remission. In effect, the individual has been cured of their depression—because the root causes of their depression have been discovered and addressed.

Stripes of the zebra

One way I like to think about biochemical individuality is to think about zebras.

Since childhood, I have been fascinated by these sensitive, powerful creatures. Zebras, I learned, have acute senses, to instantly alert them to nearby predators. To avoid those predators, they move in a zigzag pattern. And they have plenty of stamina to outlast the carnivores that pursue them.

But the most interesting thing I learned about zebras—animals that seem to look pretty much alike at first glance—is that each one of them has a unique pattern of stripes, like a fingerprint.

There are black zebras with white stripes, the standard issue. But some have brown stripes. Some have black stripes. Some have black *and* white stripes.

Some stripes are narrow. Some are broad. Some cover the zebra's legs, and some don't. Some cover the belly, and some don't. Some stripes are more vertical, some more horizontal. Some have sharp edges, some blurry.

Bottom line (or maybe bottom stripe):

In nature, individuality—not homogeneity—is the rule.

And for effective treatment, taking individuality into account is a must.

Yes, the symptoms of depression are similar enough from person to person that mental health professionals have created the well-defined diagnostic categories of depression, like "major depressive disorder" and "postpartum depression" and so on.

But the *causes* of those symptoms are as diverse as the stripes of the zebra. Diverse enough to require personalized, precision medicine, one of the hallmarks of Functional Psychiatry.

Which leads me to my next point.

Treating causes, not symptoms

I've said this many times already in this chapter, but it's so important I'm going to say it again:

Conventional psychiatric medicine treats *symptoms*.

Functional Psychiatry discovers and treats *root causes*.

Think of the difference between attending to symptoms and causes as something like this:

If the oil light on the dashboard of your car goes on, you can shoot out the light—that is, get rid of the symptom.

Or you can conduct diagnostic tests to figure out what's *causing* the low oil light to go on. An oil leak. The need for an oil change. A failed oil pump. A failed oil pressure sensor. Engine damage. Etc. And once you've found the cause, you can actually correct the problem.

"The Tomato Effect"

Why nutritional therapies are rejected by mainstream medicine

Everybody knows that tomatoes are bad for you, right? In fact, they're *poisonous*. Take one bite, and you'll be sick in minutes. Eat an entire tomato, and you'll probably be dead.

Well, this seemingly absurd idea—that tomatoes are the botanical equivalent of cyanide—was commonly believed in America, from the 1600s to the early nineteenth century.

It's not that fear of the so-called "poison apple" (native to Peru; imported to Spain; and quickly spread in the sixteenth century to Italy and France) was wholly without basis. Tomatoes are nightshades, a family of plants that includes potatoes, eggplants, and bell peppers. It also includes very toxic plants, like belladonna, henbane, and mandrake.

But while Americans were avoiding tomatoes like the plague, Europeans were happily consuming the plant—in pizza, sauces, soups, and other dishes. And here's the strangest part of the story.

New World Americans *knew* that their old-world brethren had been chowing down on tomatoes for centuries without any ill effects. But they refused to believe the vegetable was safe for human consumption!

That situation changed in 1820, when a brave soul named Robert Gibbon Johnson—a historian and horticulturist—publicly ate a basket of tomatoes on the steps of the Old Salem County Courthouse in New Jersey. And lived to tell the tale.

Over the next century, tomatoes were cultivated in more and more American farms and backyards—and became a standard of the American diet. (Americans now eat about thirty pounds per year, second only to potatoes.)

Rejecting effective therapies

I'm telling you this story because it perfectly illustrates a medical frame of mind that has been aptly dubbed "the tomato effect"—the rejection of highly effective therapies because they don't fit with the prevailing belief system.

In an editorial in the *Journal of the American Medical Association* titled "The Tomato Effect," the husband-and-wife team of Dr. James Goodwin (internal medicine) and Dr. Jean Goodwin (psychiatry) wrote:

> "The tomato effect in medicine occurs when an efficacious treatment for a certain disease is ignored or rejected because it does not 'make sense' in light of the accepted theories of disease mechanism and drug interaction.
>
> "The tomato was ignored because it was clearly poisonous; it would have been foolish to eat one. In analogous fashion, there have been many therapies in the history of medicine that, while later proved highly efficacious, were at one time rejected because they did not make sense."[5]

Later in the editorial, the Drs. Goodwin make a point that I think is particularly relevant to targeted nutritional supplementation for depression and other types of mental illness:

> "In this atmosphere we are at risk for rejecting a safe, inexpensive, effective therapy in favor of a treatment perhaps less efficacious and more toxic."

This is exactly what has happened with nutritional supplementation for mental illness.

Understanding this very human tendency to reject a treatment outside of one's frame of reference—even in the presence of contradictory evidence—helps us identify *why* the medical profession has resisted the importance of nutritional deficiencies and imbalances in brain function.

Participating in the paradigm shift

But that resistance is softening—even melting—with the advent of Functional Psychiatry. The old medical model is giving way to a new one.

This "paradigm shift"—a term coined by historian of science Thomas Kuhn, PhD, in his influential book *The Structure of*

Scientific Revolutions—is happening because of several factors. Kuhn specifies three of them:

Evidence to the contrary. There is an accumulation of evidence showing that nutritional deficiencies and imbalances are a leading factor in mental illness and health. In fact, the literature is vast—with thousands of studies demonstrating that deficiencies in nutrients like omega-3 fatty acids, B vitamins, vitamin D, and zinc (to name a few) are linked to mental health disorders. Because of this research, more clinicians are questioning the validity of the current paradigm, and exploring new avenues of treatment.

Education. The training of clinicians and researchers with a fresh perspective and approach can contribute to a paradigm shift.

Social and cultural factors. Patients like you—the society and culture of those with mental disorders—are leading the way, too. They are literally sick and tired of an ineffective medical paradigm for treating mental illness. They are fed up with a theory and practice that doesn't work. They are weary of an approach to mental disorders that ignores the imbalanced biology underlying the disorder, and instead focuses on treating symptoms. They want change. They want *healing*. My hope is that Functional Psychiatry can help provide that change, improving the mental health and well-being of thousands of patients.

In other words, we can all start eating and enjoying "tomatoes"—targeted nutritional supplementation for better mental health.

Conventional medicine tends to shoot out the oil light.

Functional Psychiatry finds and fixes the underlying problem.

You are not to blame for your depression

Functional Psychiatry is not interested in assigning the "blame" for your depression on your past, or on some character flaw.

This stigmatization of the depressed is wrong!

Depression is a medical condition, not a weakness.

There is no one to blame. There is only a rational, multistep process that 1) acknowledges the deficiencies and imbalanced biochemistry that affects the brain; 2) identifies the deficiencies and imbalances; 3) treats the deficiencies and imbalances; 4) achieves a healthier brain; and 5) reduces or resolves depression.

Let's take a look at how Functional Psychiatry helped one of my depressed patients—ending five years of dismal suffering.

The Story of Frank:
After Five Years of Depression—
Depression Free!

Frank was fifty years old when he decided that he needed to find a different approach to treating his long-standing depressive symptoms.

For five years, Frank had been struggling with low mood and fatigue. He'd gone to his primary care provider, who had listened sympathetically, and prescribed an antidepressant. The medication had only minimal benefits, so the doctor tried switching Frank to a different medication—which also didn't provide much relief. At that point, the primary care doctor referred Frank to a psychiatrist.

Frank had assumed he'd easily find relief, now that he was being treated by a mental health specialist. But all the psychiatrist did was continue the antidepressant—and prescribe *more* medications, including an antipsychotic and an antianxiety drug.

Not surprisingly, the depression continued. And now Frank was also dealing with troublesome side effects from the medications, like weight gain and erectile dysfunction.

Frank heard from a friend about my practice of Functional Psychiatry, and made an appointment.

As I took his medical history, Frank told me his sex drive was low, and that he'd slowly but surely gained weight. He said he had a poor sense of taste, and gravitated toward greasy, salty junk food. He also told me that he never felt rested upon awakening—he started his day tired. And his mouth was very dry in the morning, like he'd been sucking on sand. Finally, he told me that his wife complained about how much he snored over the course of a night. The history also revealed Frank had no familial history of mental illness.

As you read earlier in this chapter, a key step in the process of Functional Psychiatry is *testing*.

I ordered comprehensive laboratory testing (including the ION Profile from Genova Diagnostics, which analyzes more than 125 nutrient biomarkers), and also a sleep study, to determine if Frank had sleep apnea, a type of breathing difficulty during sleep that causes daytime fatigue—and raises the risk of depression.

The results were telling:

Low testosterone. Frank's total testosterone was very low, at 193 nanograms per deciliter (ng/dL), and his free testosterone was also low, at 22 ng/dL.

In middle-aged men like Frank, testosterone that low is nearly a guarantee for low energy, low libido, and low mood (not to mention low confidence and low focus). Low testosterone also encourages abdominal fat.

Low zinc. Blood levels of zinc were low. As you'll read in Chapter 7, studies show that low zinc levels are strongly linked to depression, and that supplementing with zinc can help treat depression. In fact, some researchers say that zinc is an accurate biomarker for depression: The lower the zinc, the more depressive symptoms you're likely to have.

Sleep apnea. The sleep study showed Frank had mild to moderate sleep apnea, which can triple the risk for depression.

After testing, treatment

I had tested Frank. Now it was time to treat him.

Testosterone replacement therapy. Frank received testosterone replacement therapy, with regular injections.

Zinc supplementation. He took 30 milligrams (mg) of zinc picolinate daily.

Continuous positive airway pressure (CPAP), for sleep apnea. He started using CPAP treatment, a gold-standard treatment for sleep apnea, helping keep the airways open during sleep.

I made a follow-up appointment for two months later.

"Mostly recovered"

When Frank returned to my office after two months, he said—remarkably—that he was feeling "mostly recovered" from depression.

Let's pause for a second to think about what had just happened.

This middle-aged man had been struggling with nonstop depression for *five years*. He had taken three antidepressants and other psychoactive medications, all to *no* effect. Yes, he was diagnosed with "depression"—but he had *never* been tested for any of its underlying biological causes. Yet, once that testing was done, and the causes identified and treated—Frank recovered in only two months!

In the practice of Functional Psychiatry, that type of outstanding result is not miraculous—it is commonplace. Or maybe it's more accurate to say, in Functional Psychiatry, the seemingly miraculous *is* commonplace.

And there was even more good news for Frank.

After two months, he had no more morning fatigue, and his daytime energy was much improved. I attributed that to the CPAP, which helped him overcome his sleep apnea, and sleep more deeply.

With the testosterone supplementation, his sex drive increased, which (needless to say) had a positive effect on his relationship with his wife.

Another big plus: The mineral zinc plays a key role in the sense of taste—and zinc supplementation had restored Frank's ability to taste (and enjoy) foods. He told me that he found it much easier to make healthy food choices, because whole foods had more flavor.

He also told me that he thought both the testosterone and zinc had gone a long way toward improving his mood and his sense of well-being.

Frank's case is a perfect example of the power of functional medicine to overcome depression.

Frank had *not* responded to five different psychoactive medications.

But by taking a step back and identifying the factors that were the possible *causes* of Frank's symptoms, we could personalize a treatment approach—and resolve Frank's depression.

Functional Psychiatry can do the same for you. And you can start *now*, without any testing whatsoever, using the Essential Functional Psychiatry Treatment Plan.

Start with the Essential Functional Psychiatry Treatment Plan

I've distilled the core nutritional treatments of this book into a simple protocol that *anyone* can use for three months—without testing. It features the targeted nutritional supplements discussed in Part II, where you can read a wealth of information about each of these nutrients: what they are; how and why they work; scientific evidence supporting their use; and stories of people who have benefited by using them. This "Essential" plan consists of eight supplements:

Free-form amino acids. This supplement, which you can read about in Chapter 4, balances neurotransmitters, often producing remarkably positive results—better mood and more energy—within weeks. It is often the cornerstone of my treatment plans for a patient with depression. **Dose:** Take one scoop (4 grams, or g) twice daily, in a glass of water or juice between meals. I recommend the product Free-Form Amino Acids, from Pure Encapsulations. (Pure Encapsulations is the number one doctor-used brand of nutritional supplements, and I consistently prescribe them—and recommend them—because of their reliability and effectiveness.) Don't mix with a protein-rich liquid, like yogurt or milk, which will decrease absorption.

Vitamin D. Low levels of this nutrient, which you can read about in Chapter 5, are strongly linked to depression. **Dose:** 2,000 international units (IU) daily, in a supplement that also contains vitamin K2. **Important:** You can start this nutrient without laboratory testing, but eventual testing is a must. Long-term, you need to discover your blood level and take a dosage that reliably boosts your vitamin D to an optimal level.

Vitamin B complex. Low levels of many B vitamins—particularly folate and vitamin B12, which you can read about in Chapter 6—play a role in depression. **Dose:** Taking a vitamin B complex supplement can supply adequate doses of all the B vitamins. I recommend the product B-Complex Plus, from Pure Encapsulations. (The form of folate in this supplement—L-methylfolate [LMF]—bypasses a common genetic mutation that blocks the absorption of folic acid.) Follow the dosage recommendation on the label. **Important:** You can start this supplement without laboratory testing. But, as Chapter 6 explains at length, there are several laboratory tests that are crucial in determining your individualized therapeutic dose of vitamin B12.

Trace mineral supplement. Zinc, chromium, iodine, and several other trace minerals, which you can read about in Chapter 7, are vital in brain health and in preventing and treating depression. **Dose:** A single trace mineral supplement can supply therapeutic doses of all the key trace minerals. I recommend Trace Minerals from Pure Encapsulations. Follow the dosage recommendation on the label.

Magnesium. This mineral, which you can read about in Chapter 7, plays a role in hundreds of biochemical processes in the body, including in the brain, and is a must for mental health and positive mood. Magnesium also relaxes muscles and nerves, and aids sleep. **Dose:** 240 mg daily (120 mg, twice a day, at breakfast and before bed). I recommend magnesium glycinate.

Lithium orotate. Low levels of this trace mineral, which you can read about in Chapter 8, are strongly linked to depression, mood swings, and to irritability and aggression. You can take low-dose nutritional lithium in the form of lithium orotate without testing. **Dose:** I recommend 1 mg daily, from Pure Encapsulations.

Omega-3 fatty acids, EPA and DHA. These two components of fat, which you can read about in Chapter 9, are a must for neuron-to-neuron communication and treating depression. You can take an omega-3 supplement safely and effectively for three months, but I recommend testing at that point to customize the dose. **Dose:** 2 to 3 g daily of total EPA/DHA.

Curcumin and oligomeric proanthocyanidins (OPCs). The active ingredient in the spice turmeric, curcumin—which you can read about in Chapter 10—is a powerful anti-inflammatory, reducing the neuroinflammation that is linked to depression.

Found in green tea, red grapes, blueberries, and other colorful plants, OPCs—which you can also read about in Chapter 10—are also anti-inflammatory and help balance brainwaves. The product CurcumaSorb Mind from Pure Encapsulations provides therapeutic dosages of both curcumin and OPCs. Follow the dosage recommendation on the label.

That's the Essential Functional Psychiatry Treatment Plan—the essence of targeted nutritional supplementation for depression. You can safely start that plan today, without testing. However, the foundation of Functional Psychiatry *is* testing—and a personalized treatment plan based on your test results. If possible, try to get all of your testing completed *before* starting nutritional supplementation.

Essential Functional Psychiatry Treatment Plan

SUPPLEMENT	IMPORTANCE	DOSING	NOTES
Amino Replete *Pure Encapsulations*	Balances neuro-transmitters, often producing remarkable results—better mood and more energy—within weeks.	Take one scoop (4 g) twice daily in a glass of water or juice between meals.	Don't mix with a protein-rich liquid like yogurt or milk, which will decrease absorption. *Read about it in Chapter 4.*
Vitamin D3 & K2 *Pure Encapsulations*	Low levels of vitamin D are strongly linked to depression.	Take one capsule daily with food.	You can start this nutrient without laboratory testing. But long-term, testing is a must to determine your blood level of vitamin D and take a dosage that boosts the vitamin to optimal levels. *Read about it in Chapter 5.*
B-Complex Plus *Pure Encapsulations*	Low levels of many B vitamins—particularly folate and vitamin B12—play a role in depression.	Take one capsule, once or twice daily with food.	You can start a B complex supplement without laboratory testing. Long-term, however, laboratory testing is necessary to determine the individualized dose of vitamin B12 that is right for you. *Read about it in Chapter 6.*
Trace Minerals *Pure Encapsulations*	Zinc, chromium, iodine, and several other trace minerals are vital for brain health and in preventing and treating depression.	Take one capsule, once or twice daily with food.	A single trace mineral supplement can supply therapeutic doses of all the key trace minerals. *Read about it in Chapter 7.*
Magnesium Glycinate *Pure Encapsulations*	Magnesium plays a role in hundreds of biochemical processes in the body, including in the brain, and is a must for supporting mental health.	Take 240 mg daily: 120 mg, twice a day, at breakfast and before bed.	Magnesium relaxes the muscles and nerves, and aids sleep. *Read about it in Chapter 7.*

SUPPLEMENT	IMPORTANCE	DOSING	NOTES
Lithium (orotate) *Pure Encapsulations*	Low intake of this trace mineral is strongly linked to suicidality (thinking about or attempting suicide), irritability, and aggression.	Take 2 mg daily.	You can take 1 or 2 mg of low-dose nutritional lithium (lithium orotate) daily without testing. However, do not take more than 10 mg without the guidance of a doctor experienced in the use of low-dose nutritional lithium. *Read about it in Chapter 8.*
Equazen *SFI Health*	This product has a three-to-one ratio of EPA to DHA, which are components of fat that help neuron-to-neuron communication and treat depression.	Take three to six softgels daily with meals.	You can take an omega-3 supplement without testing for three months. But testing at that point is highly recommended to determine the right dose for you. *Read about it in Chapter 9.*
CurcumaSorb Mind *Pure Encapsulations*	Curcumin, the active ingredient in the spice turmeric, is a powerful anti-inflammatory, reducing the neuroinflammation that is often linked to depression.	Take two capsules, one to three times daily between meals.	The OPCs found in green tea, red grapes, blueberries, and other colorful plants have a wide variety of brain-healing effects, including balancing the levels of several neurotransmitters. *Read about it in Chapter 10.*

CHAPTER 3

First Test, Then Treat

Using testing to discover your unique imbalances and deficiencies is the missing link in effectively treating depression.

Functional Psychiatry takes a new, more comprehensive approach to finding and fixing the causes of depression. As I emphasize throughout the book: the latest scientific research shows that depression (and other mental health problems) is often caused or complicated by underlying imbalances in the body, including nutrient deficiencies, inflammation, chronic infections, disturbances in gut bacteria, and many others.

By *finding* and then *fixing* these imbalances—by first *testing* and then *treating*—Functional Psychiatry is able to create personalized protocols for overcoming depression, rather than the "one-size-fits-all" approach of taking an antidepressant medication. Using testing as the foundation, Functional Psychiatry acknowledges, discovers, and addresses your *biochemical individuality*, the unique constellation of imbalances that underlies and sustains your depression.

This use of objective laboratory-based diagnostics is hardly an anomaly in medicine. Doctors do this with most health problems! Case in point:

Imagine a patient showing up at their primary care physician's office with chest pain. But instead of using objective testing to find out the underlying cause of the pain, the physician does nothing but listen to the patient describe their subjective symptoms—and then prescribes a medication like a statin or a blood thinner.

Needless to say, that's a far cry from "gold-standard" medicine for chest pain. In fact, prescribing a drug without accompanying objective testing would be considered malpractice in the diagnosis and treatment of chest pain. Anyone with chest pain is likely to get a range of tests, like an electrocardiogram (ECG), a chest X-ray, and blood tests for heart biomarkers like troponins (to detect a heart attack).

But as I said a moment ago, many medical doctors, including many psychiatrists, take a subjective approach with depression—they don't recognize depression can and often does have underlying *biological* causes.

And once these underlying biological causes have been identified through objective testing, you and your doctor can use the test results to develop a *personalized* treatment plan to correct imbalances—with targeted nutritional supplementation and diet; with lifestyle changes; with therapy; with medications; and with many other therapeutic approaches.

This approach—the approach of Functional Psychiatry—is the road to relief and lasting recovery. A road you can travel with the map provided by this book.

A simple case history highlights the benefits of lab tests and their objective results.

Mary, a woman in her late twenties, had been dealing with depression and fatigue for nearly a decade. She had been prescribed numerous medications and received years of counseling, all without much benefit.

When she first walked into my office, I immediately noticed how pale she looked. An initial round of testing showed that her complete blood count (CBC) was normal—that is, she had normal levels of red blood cells (low levels signal a possible iron deficiency).

But another round of testing revealed she had very low ferritin levels, a measure of stored iron. Her body had compensated for her low iron levels by maintaining red blood cell formation. But she still had numerous symptoms linked to iron deficiency—including chronic depression and fatigue!

Over the next few months, iron supplementation dramatically improved her depression symptoms.

She was tested. She was treated. And she healed.

Tests to Consider

Throughout this book, I recommend many different tests, depending on the biological imbalance—the root cause—that I'm discussing in a particular chapter. Homocysteine testing for a suspected B vitamin deficiency (Chapter 6). Trace Mineral Hair Analysis to detect mineral deficiencies (Chapter 7).

It's highly unlikely you're going to want to get every test covered in this book. To help you and your doctor decide which tests are best for you, I've created this at-a-glance guide to nearly two dozen objective tests for depression. Some of the key considerations when thinking about ordering any test:

- Do you need this test? That is, is the test not only important, but important for *you*? As you'll see, every test discussed in this chapter includes a list of factors which, if they apply to you, indicate you should probably *prioritize* that particular test.

- Does the test require a doctor's orders, or can you order it yourself? Does insurance typically cover it?

- What is the best way to interpret results to help you overcome depression?

But before you start reading about the tests themselves, here are a few caveats and cautions.

What is normal? For each test, I've indicated a value that shows if your results are normal. But laboratory testing isn't that straightforward. Labs frequently develop their own values based on results from the people they've already tested, creating discrepancies from lab to lab. And as I explain in other chapters, even so-called "normal" results (for B12 levels, for example) may require treatment.

False results. Tests results are occasionally incorrect, with a "false positive" (the results say your values are normal, but they're not) or a "false negative" (the results say your values are out of the normal range, but they're not).

One test is not the answer. Don't consider any test in isolation. Look at *all* your results and *then* create a protocol that makes sense.

Partner with a health care professional. If at all possible, I strongly recommend you work with a qualified health care provider, like a primary care physician, psychiatrist, or naturopathic doctor familiar with Functional Medicine. They are very likely to have the training and expertise to help you interpret and act upon your test results.

All that said, here are the most important tests I use in my practice. I've organized them in order of importance—that is, I start with the tests of "High Importance" that are *most likely* to detect a previously hidden cause of depression that you and your health care provider can then correct, and proceed from there, to tests of "Moderate" and "Low" importance.

Celiac screening

I can't emphasize enough the importance of this test because undetected celiac disease—which causes many nutritional deficiencies—underlies many cases of depression.

There are several variations of this blood test. But at minimum it should measure *antitissue transglutaminase immunoglobulin a antibody* and *total immunoglobulin A (IgA)* levels. If you have celiac disease—an autoimmune disease that affects the intestinal tract—it's important to detect and treat it. (One study shows the risk of long-lasting, low-grade depression is five times higher in people with diagnosed celiac disease.) I discuss celiac disease and depression in Chapter 11.

Prioritize this test if:

- you have gastrointestinal symptoms, especially diarrhea or abdominal pain;
- you have unexplained weight loss; and/or
- you have long-standing depression that has been resistant to numerous treatments.

Doctor's orders: Direct-to-consumer testing is available.

Insurance coverage: Possible, depending on the diagnostic codes submitted with testing, such as abdominal pain, diarrhea, or abnormal weight loss.

Normal values: Negative transglutaminase IgA.

Goal for treating depression: Normal values.

Additional info: If total IgA levels are low, the transglutaminase IgA test results could be an inaccurate false negative. In that case, an antitissue transglutaminase immunoglobulin G (IgG) test is often added. Also, you need to be eating wheat or gluten on a regular basis for the test to be accurate.

Complete Blood Count (CBC)

This standard blood test provides a snapshot of your overall health by measuring key blood components like red blood cells (RBCs), white blood cells (WBCs), hemoglobin, hematocrit, and platelets.

An annual CBC test establishes a baseline for normal blood values, helping a doctor identify any worrisome deviation.

Prioritize this test if: You should receive a CBC test yearly as part of an annual health exam.

Doctor's orders: Direct-to-consumer testing is available.

Insurance coverage: Yes, typically.

Normal values: Varies, based on the test component.

Goal for treating depression: Normal laboratory values.

Comprehensive metabolic panel (CMP)

This blood test evaluates electrolytes (minerals), kidney function, liver function, acid-base balance (pH), blood sugar levels, and protein levels.

Like CBC, an annual CMP test is important for detecting any variations in the basics of metabolic health.

Prioritize this test if: You should receive a CMP test on a yearly basis as part of an annual exam.

Doctor's orders: Direct-to-consumer testing is available.

Insurance coverage: Yes, typically.

Normal values: Varies, based on the test component.

Goal for treating depression: Normal laboratory values.

Lipid panel

This blood test measures blood fats like total cholesterol, low-density lipoprotein (LDL), and triglycerides. *Low* total cholesterol is a commonly overlooked risk factor for depression and suicidality, which I discuss in Chapter 9. Additionally, depression increases the risk of heart attacks and strokes by 35 percent, so if you're depressed you want to make sure to control your risk factors for heart disease.

Prioritize this test if:

- you are suicidal or have any self-harming behaviors, like cutting;
- you struggle with aggressive or violent impulses; and/or
- you have a family history of cardiovascular disease (heart attack, heart failure, or stroke).

Doctor's orders: Direct-to-consumer testing is available.

Insurance coverage: Yes, typically.

Normal values: Total cholesterol, < 200 milligrams per deciliter (mg/dL).

Goal for treating depression: Total cholesterol, between 130 to 200 mg/dL.

Iron panel and ferritin

These blood tests include: serum iron (the amount of iron in the blood); iron-binding capacity (a measurement of how well the body can transport iron in the blood); iron saturation percentage (the amount of iron that is bound to protein carriers); and ferritin (stored iron). I discuss the importance of iron in depression in Chapter 7.

Prioritize these tests if:

- your energy levels are low;
- you are a vegan, vegetarian, or don't eat much meat;
- you have a menstrual cycle, especially if you have heavy bleeding;
- you have recent blood loss;
- A CBC test shows you have a low red blood cell (RBC) count, low hematocrit, or low hemoglobin, especially in cases where mean corpuscular volume (MCV) or mean corpuscular hemoglobin concentration (MCHC; the average concentration of hemoglobin in a given volume of RBCs) are also low.

Doctor's orders: Direct-to-consumer testing is available.

Insurance coverage: Yes, typically.

Normal values: Iron, 50–180 micrograms per deciliter (mcg/dL); iron-binding capacity, 250–425 mcg/dL; percent saturation, 20–48% ferritin, 38–380 nanograms per milliliter (ng/mL).

Goal for treating depression: Normal values (ferritin, 70–100 ng/mL).

Vitamin D (25-hydroxy vitamin D)

This blood test measures blood levels of stored vitamin D (25-hydroxy vitamin D), with low levels strongly linked to depression. (One study, for example, shows that people with a vitamin D deficiency have a 75 percent higher risk of developing depression than people with normal levels.) I discuss vitamin D in Chapter 5.

Prioritize this test if:

- you have a mental health condition;
- you don't get much sunlight (which triggers the formation of vitamin D in the body) or live in a location with a latitude 37° north or higher, like New York City, Boston, Chicago, or Seattle; or
- you are not Caucasian. (Darker-skinned people create lower levels of vitamin D.)

Doctor's orders: Direct-to-consumer testing is available.

Insurance coverage: Depends on the diagnostic codes, such as osteoporosis, chronic kidney disease, and obesity.

Normal values: 30–100 ng/mL.

Goal for treating depression: 40–60 ng/mL.

Additional info: Low levels of vitamin D are linked not only to depression and bipolar disorder but also to ADHD, schizophrenia, and other mental health conditions, as well as more severe respiratory infections, heart disease, cancer, and multiple sclerosis.

MTHFR Genetic Test

This test uses a blood draw or cheek swab to measure the genetic profile of methylenetetrahydrofolate reductase (MTHFR), an enzyme involved in *methylation*, a biochemical process that plays many roles in the body. A common genetic mutation in this enzyme (40 percent of the adult population) can block the absorption of the B vitamin folate, causing depression. I discuss the importance of MTHFR testing in Chapter 6.

Prioritize this test if:

- you have a family history of mental health problems or heart disease; or
- you have treatment-resistant depression and haven't responded well to medications.

Doctor's orders: Direct-to-consumer testing is available.

Insurance coverage: No, typically.

Normal values: Homozygous (normal) for both genetic copies of MTHFR, without C677T or A1298C mutations.

Goal for treating depression: If the test is not normal, take a methylated form of folate (L-methylfolate, or LMF), as discussed in Chapter 6.

C-reactive protein (CRP)

This test measures a biomarker of inflammation—and inflammation has been linked to depression, with one study showing that 50 percent of depressed patients had modest to significant elevations in inflammation as measured by CRP.

Prioritize this test if:

- you have chronic pain, a sign of chronic inflammation;
- you have a personal or family history of heart disease, because chronic inflammation puts you at increased risk for this disease; or
- you have an autoimmune condition, like lupus, rheumatoid arthritis, or inflammatory bowel disease.

Doctor's orders: Direct-to-consumer testing is available.

Insurance coverage: Possible, depending on the diagnostic codes submitted with testing (for example, if the diagnosis code indicates joint pain, which is often related to inflammation).

Normal values: < 1 milligrams per liter (mg/L).

Goal for treating depression: Normal values.

Additional info: There are different types of CRP testing. For the test to have better diagnostic value, choose a "highly sensitive" test, which gives numerical results.

Vitamin B12

This blood test measures vitamin B12. As I discuss in Chapter 6, a deficiency of this vitamin is common in people with depression—and correcting a deficiency is a must.

Prioritize this test if:

- you have cognitive decline;
- you have *macrocytic anemia*, a condition that includes low hemoglobin or hematocrit levels and an MCV over 100 femtoliters (fL);
- you have neuropathy, a condition that usually includes pain and tingling in the hands or feet;
- you are vegetarian, vegan, or don't consume much meat (B12 is found almost exclusively in animal products); or
- you don't eat a lot of vegetables, especially leafy greens, which are the best source of folate.

Doctor's orders: Direct-to-consumer testing is available.

Insurance coverage: Possibly, based on the diagnostic codes submitted by your doctor, like for nutritional anemia or fatigue.

Normal values (for adults): 200–1100 picograms per milliliter (pg/mL).

Goal for treating depression: >600 pg/mL.

Zinc and copper

This blood or hair test measures levels of copper and zinc, which balance each other in the body (the higher the zinc, the lower the copper, and vice versa). Low levels of zinc and high levels of copper are both linked to increased risk of depression, and zinc is effective in the treatment of depression. I discuss these two minerals and their symbiotic relationship in Chapter 7.

Prioritize this test if:

- you have a mental health problem;
- you are a vegetarian, vegan, or eat only limited amount of animal products (which are the richest source of zinc);
- you are irritable;
- you have a digestive condition that can lower zinc absorption, like celiac disease, inflammatory bowel disease, or irritable bowel syndrome (IBS); or
- you are taking a diuretic or a proton pump inhibitor (PPI), both of which lower zinc levels.

Doctor's orders: Direct-to-consumer testing is available.

Insurance coverage: No, typically.

Normal values: Varies widely by lab.

Goal for treating depression: Mid-range values for both zinc and copper.

Additional info: Another way to measure zinc is with the Zinc Taste Test (ZTT), also called the Zinc Tally Test. It's based on the idea that the ability to taste zinc sulfate varies depending on your zinc status. For the test, you hold a small amount of zinc sulfate solution in your mouth for about ten seconds. If you experience an immediate, strong metallic or bitter taste—your zinc levels are probably fine. If you have a delayed or weak taste of the zinc, you may have a marginal zinc deficiency. And if you don't taste zinc at all—if the solution tastes water-like—you may have a zinc deficiency. The test is simple, cheap, and easy to take, and is widely available. And over the many decades of my psychiatric practice, I've found it very reliable.

Thyroid panel and thyroid antibodies

The thyroid panel is a blood test that measures thyroid-stimulating hormone (TSH) and levels of free T4 and free T3, which I discuss in Chapter 12. This test detects imbalanced thyroid hormones, which are linked to depression. The thyroid antibody test is a blood test that detects thyroid antibodies like thyroid peroxidase (TPO) and antithyroglobulin (ATG), which indicate an autoimmune disease of the thyroid gland (the immune system attacks the thyroid gland as if it were a foreign invader like a virus).

Prioritize this test if:

- you have symptoms of low thyroid function, like low mood, fatigue, muscle and joint pain, constipation, and dry skin; or

- you have symptoms of hyperthyroidism, like anxiety, irritability, rapid heartbeat, unexplained weight loss, or goiter (an enlarged thyroid gland).

Doctor's orders: Direct-to-consumer testing is available.

Insurance coverage: Depends on diagnostic codes (such as thyroid disorders, and symptoms potentially related to thyroid dysfunction), and the panel components being ordered (TSH only is more likely to be approved).

Normal values: TSH, 0.4–4.5 milli-international units per liter (mIU/L). Free T4, 0.8–1.8 ng/dL. Free T3, 2.3–4.2 pg/mL. TPO, < 9 mIU/mL. Antithyroglobulin, ≤ 1mIU/mL.

Goals for treating depression: TSH, 0.4–2.5 mIU/L. Free T4, 1.3–1.8 ng/dL.

Free T3, 3.2–4.2 pg/mL. TPO, < 9 mIU/mL. Antithyroglobulin, ≤ 1 mIU/mL.

DHEA-S and pregnenolone

This is a blood, urine, or saliva test that measures dehydroepiandrosterone sulfate (DHEA-S) and pregnenolone, so-called "steroid hormones" that are precursors to other hormones, like cortisol, and the sex hormones estrogen and testosterone. Low levels of DHEA-S and pregnenolone have been linked to depression, as discussed in Chapter 12.

Prioritize this test if:

- you have an irregular menstrual cycle;
- you have symptoms of low testosterone, including erectile dysfunction; or
- your depression symptoms have been resistant to standard treatments.

Doctor's orders: Direct-to-consumer testing is available.

Insurance coverage: No, except in cases of specific conditions related to hormone levels, like polycystic ovary syndrome (PCOS).

Normal values: Depends on the lab and the sample type.

Goal for treating depression: Values in the mid-range, not low-normal or low.

Homocysteine

This blood test measures homocysteine, an amino acid that is produced by the body and converted into cysteine, another amino acid. But if the conversion is blocked, homocysteine levels can increase to toxic amounts—leading to cellular damage from oxidation and inflammation, blood clots, and heart disease. High levels of homocysteine are also linked to depression, bipolar disorder, schizophrenia, and Alzheimer's disease. And high levels of homocysteine can mean low levels of folate, and also vitamin B12, vitamin B6, and zinc. I discuss homocysteine in Chapter 6.

Prioritize this test if:

- you have migraine headaches, with aura or visual disturbances (homocysteine worsens migraines by causing inflammation, damaging blood vessels, and increasing the "excitability" of neurons);
- you have a family history of dementia, or concerns about cognitive decline;
- you have macular degeneration, an age-related eye disease that reduces vision;

- you have had a stroke; or
- you have a personal or family history of heart disease.

Doctor's orders: Direct-to-consumer testing is available.

Insurance coverage: Possibly, depending on the diagnostic codes used for ordering the test, such as high blood pressure, type 2 diabetes, and folate deficiency anemia.

Normal values: Male, < 11.4 micromoles per liter (μmol/L); female, < 10.4 μmol/L.

Goal for treating depression: 7–9 μmol/L.

RBC toxic and nutrient minerals

This blood test detects the level of about twenty minerals in red blood cells (RBCs), from toxic minerals like arsenic to essential minerals like zinc and magnesium.

Prioritize this test if:

- you have a poor diet, or suspect toxic chemicals are causing health problems.

Doctor's orders: Yes, typically.

Insurance coverage: No, typically.

Normal values: Varies per mineral and by laboratory.

Goal for treating depression: For nutritional minerals—like calcium, iron, magnesium, selenium, and zinc—normal to upper normal ranges. For toxic metals—like mercury, lead, cadmium, aluminum, and arsenic—as low as possible.

Urinary organic acids

This urine test measures organic acids, byproducts of metabolism. Of particular importance is 3-hydroxypropionic acid (HPHPA), a metabolic byproduct of certain bacteria in the gut that can disrupt neurotransmitter function—and trigger depression (and other types of mental health problems, like ADHD).

Prioritize this test if:

- you have depression, ADHD, schizophrenia, autism, or obsessive-compulsive disorder.

Doctor's orders: Yes, typically (for the most accurate results, work with a doctor familiar with this test).

Insurance coverage: No, typically.

Normal values: Depends on the lab conducting the test.

Goal for treating depression: Values within the normal range listed on the lab report.

Additional info: Many different organic acids are linked to mental health problems. High levels of methylmalonic acid (MMA) can indicate a vitamin B12 deficiency, which can trigger depression. High levels of kynurenate can indicate low levels of B6, also linked to depression.

Lithium

This hair or urine test measures lithium, a mineral strongly linked to depression, suicidality, and bipolar disorder. I consider low-dose nutritional lithium so important in the treatment of depression that I devote an entire chapter to it (Chapter 8).

You can take low-dose nutritional lithium without testing, up to 10 mg daily.

Prioritize this test if:

- you have a family history of mental health problems;
- you struggle with and/or have a family history of addiction;
- you have symptoms of irritability, like frequently feeling frustrated, impatient, and hostile (such as road rage); or
- you are suicidal, or have any self-harming behaviors.

Doctor's orders: Direct-to-consumer testing is available.

Insurance coverage: No, typically.

Normal values: For hair, 0.007–0.02 micrograms per gram (µg/g).

Goal for treating depression: Upper range of normal values.

Hormones (estrogen, progesterone, and testosterone)

There are various blood tests to measure these hormones in men and women. I discuss the link between these hormones and depression in Chapter 12.

Prioritize this test if:

- you have an irregular menstrual cycle or symptoms around the menstrual cycle;
- your libido is low;
- you are a man with gynecomastia (enlargement of breast tissue) or a woman with masculinization (including increased facial hair growth); or
- you have erectile dysfunction (ED).

Doctor's orders: Direct-to-consumer testing is available.

Insurance coverage: Possibly, depending on the diagnostic codes used for the testing, such as ED in men and PCOS in women.

Normal values: Highly variable, based on age, sex, and for women of childbearing age, the time of their menstrual cycle. Discuss with a primary care physician or endocrinologist.

Goal for treating depression: Highly variable. Discuss with a primary care physician or endocrinologist.

Kryptopyrrole testing

Kryptopyrroles are compounds that play a role in several important molecules, like hemoglobin, vitamin B12, and bile. Some individuals have high levels of kryptopyrroles, which bind with vitamin B6 and zinc, forcing these nutrients out of the body. This urine test measures kryptopyrroles in the urine. High levels of kryptopyrroles can be neurotoxic and have been linked to depression. I discuss kryptopyrroles and depression in Chapters 1 and 17.

Prioritize this test if:

- you feel easily overwhelmed by stress;
- you're an emotionally sensitive individual; or
- your skin is resistant to tanning.

Doctor's orders: Direct-to-consumer testing is available.

Normal values: 0–10 mcg/dL.

Goal for treating depression: normal values.

Amino acid panel

This test measures the amount of amino acids in your blood or urine. I discuss the importance of supplementing with "free-form amino acids" in Chapter 4.

I supplement with free-form amino acids without testing—a remarkably effective treatment that often provides rapid benefits for depressive symptoms, sometimes within days.

Prioritize this test if:

- your diet is low in protein;
- your digestion is poor, with symptoms like abdominal discomfort, bloating, constipation, and/or diarrhea; or
- you have an autoimmune disease or fibromyalgia.

Doctor's orders: Yes, typically.

Insurance coverage: No, typically.

Normal values: Varies by amino acid.

Goal for treating depression: Normal values.

Additional info: Forty-eight hours before testing, stop all supplements that contain amino acids and the artificial sweetener aspartame.

Essential fatty acids (EFAs)

As I discuss in Chapter 9, the omega-3 EFAs eicosapentaenoic acid (EPA) and docosahexaenoic acid (DHA) are a key component of brain structure and function. They also reduce inflammation, a common factor in depression. Bottom line: If you have a deficiency of omega-3 fatty acids, you're at higher risk for depression.

I supplement with omega-3s for three months without testing. After that, it's best to get a test to determine if the dose is working to boost blood levels.

Prioritize this test if:

- you have chronic pain, autoimmune conditions, or excess inflammation;
- you have a family history of dementia or Parkinson's disease, or you're concerned about cognitive decline; or
- your diet is low in seafood, a good source of omega-3s.

Doctor's orders: Direct-to-consumer testing is available.

Insurance coverage: No, typically.

Normal values: Values should be in the middle or upper half of the reference range for EPA and DHA.

Goal for treating depression: Normal values.

Magnesium

This blood test measures levels of the mineral magnesium, which I discuss in Chapter 7. The test is not that useful, however, because only 1 percent of the magnesium in the body is circulating in the bloodstream. Your results might be normal, and you could still be deficient in magnesium—and at greater risk for depression. (Testing levels of minerals like magnesium in red blood cells can help increase the accuracy of magnesium testing.)

Prioritize this test if:

- you have symptoms that indicate low magnesium levels, like constipation, muscle cramps or spasms, twitching or tremors, headaches or migraines, sleep problems, or irregular heartbeat.

Doctor's orders: Direct-to-consumer testing is available.

Insurance coverage: Possibly, depending on the diagnostic codes, such as arrythmias, electrolyte imbalances, or diabetes.

Normal values: 1.5–2.5 mg/dL.

Goal for treating depression: >2.0 mg/dL.

PART TWO

NUTRITIONAL HEALING

CHAPTER 4

Amino Acids

The Spark Plugs of Neurotransmission

> In many cases, supplementing with
> amino acids is *the* answer to depression.

want to state my position on amino acids very plainly, so it's unambiguous:

Amino acids—the precursors to neurotransmitters—
are among the most powerful antidepressants
in the medicine cabinet of Functional Psychiatry.

Amino acids can elevate mood and increase energy—and do it fast.

These effects are often dramatic, with patients describing a night-and-day difference in mood when they start supplementing with amino acids.

Amino acids feature *none* of the side effects of antidepressants. Just the opposite—they can help lessen side effects, as you'll read in Chapter 17.

I have seen so many depressed patients whose mood improved dramatically when they were given an amino acid supplement.

In fact, in my clinical practice as a Functional Psychiatrist, I have found that adding a supplement called "free-form amino acids" to the diet is sometimes the *first and only* treatment necessary to relieve depression.

If you're suffering from depression, that may sound unbelievable. If there's such a simple remedy—a single supplement—why hasn't your doctor told you about it? Well, it's very likely your doctor doesn't *know* about the supplemental use of free-form amino acids—because most doctors don't learn about the vital connection between nutrition and the health of the brain. Truth be told, many doctors are even biased against nutritional solutions, preferring the prescription pad over the pantry. But I'm pretty sure that when you learn the simple, stunning, and science-backed details of why amino acids are so uniquely powerful in lifting the fog of depression, it will make perfect (and practical) sense.

Treatment with amino acids certainly made sense to my depressed patient Maria.

The Story of Maria: Total Relief in One Month

Maria was a thirty-six-year-old woman who had been in talk therapy for a while. She'd had a stressful childhood but had been a very productive and healthy adult until she started having symptoms of fatigue and depression, with some insomnia.

Her primary care physician did blood work—complete blood count (CBC), thyroid tests, and the like—and found nothing wrong. But Maria continued to feel terrible and increasingly depressed.

In a follow-up, her primary care doctor prescribed the antidepressant Lexapro (escitalopram), without any benefit. Abilify (aripiprazole) was then added, an antipsychotic that is approved for the augmentation of the antidepressant. For her poor sleep, Ativan (lorazepam) was prescribed.

So before Maria was referred to a psychiatrist, she was already on three psychotropic medications—and not feeling any better. But a psychiatrist added two more drugs. That's not surprising, really, because it's a common practice in my field to add a couple of different medications rather than stop one that might not be helpful.

A couple of months into treatment, Maria was not any better, so Lamictal (lamotrigine), a mood stabilizer, was added. Now on six drugs, Maria came to me and said, "I'm taking all these drugs that are supposed to help me, but I feel *worse*."

The polypharmacy approach based on symptoms had failed Maria terribly. I did routine blood work, including checking her B12 and iron levels, checking her thyroid function, testing for celiac disease, etc. One result stood out: blood level of several amino acids were dramatically low. Maria had low levels of the amino acids tryptophan, phenylalanine, and tyrosine—despite the fact that she was eating a healthy diet, including plenty of protein.

My clinical experience told me that a patient with low levels of essential amino acids would have trouble making sufficient levels of neurotransmitters in the brain—and an optimal level of neurotransmitters is key to mental health and stability.

Why did Maria have low levels of amino acids?

The simple reason: poor digestion and absorption.

For her Functional Psychiatry Treatment Plan, I gave Maria: 1) absorption-improving digestive enzymes with hydrochloric acid (the stomach acid that is also a must for digestion); and 2) an amino acid formula made from free-form amino acids, for easy absorption.

In just two weeks on digestive enzymes, hydrochloric acid, and free-form amino acids, Maria felt better. After four weeks, she was back to herself.

Total relief—in one month. The same remarkable results are possible for you.

The Building Blocks of Mind and Mood

Amino acids are the building blocks of protein. And proteins, in turn, are the basic building blocks of the entire body, providing structure for skin, repairing muscle and bone, and supporting every system, organ, tissue, and cell. In fact, the main job of DNA—the informational blueprint of the body—is encoding amino acids to form the more than fifty thousand proteins that do the work of keeping you alive (and, hopefully, well).

But amino acids and proteins don't provide only *structure* to the body. They also provide *function*.

Proteins form *enzymes*, the spark plugs that activate every chemical process in the body.

Proteins form *immune molecules*, the guardians of your health against foreign invaders like viruses and bacteria.

Proteins form *hormones*, the chemical envoys of the endocrine system, which regulate every other system in the body, including the central nervous system (the spinal cord and the brain).

And amino acids form *neurotransmitters*, the brain chemicals that relay messages from one brain cell (neuron) to the next. Many antidepressants work by balancing levels of key neurotransmitters. But antidepressant medications aren't the only way to regulate neurotransmitters.

Therapeutic levels of amino acids have a similar mechanism of action, boosting your supply of serotonin and many other crucial neurotransmitters—thereby restoring balanced brain function and positive mood.

Bottom line: Amino acids can be used
as a *natural* antidepressant, with a mechanism
of action similar to antidepressant drugs
but without the burden of side effects.

Amino Acids: An Anti-Depression Primer

Amino acids are twenty-one molecules that contain carbon, hydrogen, oxygen, and nitrogen in unique configurations—and these twenty-one molecules are strung together to form the tens of thousands of proteins that power the body.

There are three types of amino acids:

Essential, because it's essential you ingest them in your daily diet for normal functioning of the body.

Conditionally essential, because they are produced by the body, but their formation can be blocked by problems like severe stress or malnutrition.

Nonessential, because they are synthesized by most cells, without any action on your part.

For energizing neurotransmission and beating depression, the three most important amino acids are phenylalanine, tryptophan, and tyrosine. 5-hydroxytryptophan (5-HTP)—a biochemical the body makes from tryptophan—is also important in boosting serotonin.

Let's look at the antidepressant power of those four compounds, one by one.

Phenylalanine: very rewarding

The essential amino acid *phenylalanine* helps create *dopamine*, the neurotransmitter that (among many other functions) controls the body's "reward center," which delivers feelings of deep satisfaction.

Additionally, phenylalanine helps create norepinephrine (also called noradrenaline), a neurotransmitter that increases alertness and focus, and controls the body's "fight-or-flight" response to stress. When you don't overreact to stress—when you're not experiencing chronic frustration and irritation—depression is less likely.

You've probably heard of *endorphins*, the feel-good brain chemicals that reduce stress, improve mood, and ease pain. (They're actually hormones that bind to opiate receptors in the brain.) There are many ways to stimulate the production of endorphins, like exercise, sex, or an enjoyable meal. But phenylalanine does it too, because it blocks the destruction of endorphins, increasing their levels.

Studies show that depressed people have lower levels of phenylalanine metabolites compared to healthy people.[1] In a study of fourteen depressed people who were given phenylethylamine—a compound derived from phenylalanine—"mood improved rapidly" in twelve of the patients, who also had "sustained antidepressant effects" for the next twenty to fifty weeks.[2]

Tyrosine: setting your body's speed limit

One more role for phenylalanine: aiding the production of *tyrosine*, an amino acid that passes easily through the "blood-brain barrier," a border of cells that stops toxins and poisons from entering the brain. Once in the brain, tyrosine is converted to dopamine, norepinephrine (noradrenaline), and epinephrine (adrenaline).

Too little tyrosine leads to low levels of dopamine, which can contribute to addictive behaviors like substance abuse.

Too little tyrosine leads to low levels of the hormones norepinephrine and epinephrine, which can contribute to stress-related depression.

Tyrosine is also the precursor to *thyroxine*, a thyroid hormone that controls the speed or "rate" of many functions in your body, like heart rate and digestion. Think of thyroxine as the accelerator and the brake pedals in your body's vehicle—if they're not working right, it's pretty likely you'll crash! In depression, your "speed" can be too slow, resulting in fatigue and little motivation. Tyrosine can help you reset your physical and emotional pace. In fact, it's very likely you need more tyrosine if you have depression and low energy.

Tryptophan and 5-HTP: serotonin suppliers

Tryptophan is the precursor to *serotonin* in the brain, an absolute requirement in the step-by-step process of its formation.

Tryptophan also makes melatonin, a hormone that helps regulate circadian rhythms, your body's alignment (or misalignment) with the daily cycle of light and dark. A "body clock" that isn't set correctly can hamper health in many ways—including low mood.

Now and then, I recommend a brief course of 1 to 2 grams (g) of tryptophan before bedtime to help with insomnia. However, I rarely recommend a tryptophan supplement for depression. That's because the brain has a tryptophan-regulating feedback mechanism that blocks the uptake of large amounts of the amino acid.

Instead, I recommend 5-HTP, another molecule in the biochemical chain that produces serotonin. 5-HTP, an extract from the seeds of the

Griffonia plant, a shrub found in West and central Africa, passes readily into the brain and is easily converted to serotonin.

Research shows that supplementing the diet with 5-HTP boosts serotonin and helps relieve depression. In a study from India, psychiatrists gave either 5-HTP or Prozac (fluoxetine) to seventy people who were experiencing their "first depressive episode." Both therapeutic agents worked equally well, with significant decreases in depression, starting two weeks after treatment and persisting for the whole eight weeks of the study. "The therapeutic efficacy of 5-HTP was considered as equal to that of fluoxetine," concluded the researchers, in the *Asian Journal of Psychiatry*.[3]

One symptom of depression that often prompts me to recommend 5-HTP is excessive rumination: repetitive, near-constant thinking about problems and negative events, in the past, present, or imagined future.

Also of interest: in animal and human studies, depression is routinely *induced* by having people at risk of depression consume a beverage meant to quickly deplete tryptophan (and serotonin). What better evidence that this amino acid is crucial to the management of depression?

Suggested dose. If you take 5-HTP, start *slowly*, taking the recommended dosage—50 to 200 milligrams (mg)—in divided doses. That's because 5-HTP can cause stomach upset, gas, and cramping. For example, if you're taking 200 mg daily, take 100 mg with two meals (breakfast and dinner).

Many clinicians also find that combining 5-HTP with tyrosine is effective. Tyrosine should also be taken in divided doses, of about 500 mg each.

But here are two very important cautions: If you're taking an antidepressant, you shouldn't take 5-HTP, tyrosine—or any individual amino acids—without your doctor's approval and guidance. The combination of 5-HTP and serotonin-boosting antidepressants like selective serotonin reuptake inhibitors (SSRIs) raises the risk of serotonin syndrome, with symptoms that range from mild (like restlessness) to life-threatening. And a person with a history of bipolar illness can become very anxious and agitated on the supplement, whether or not they're taking antidepressant medication.

More pieces of the puzzle

There are other connections between amino acids and depression.

Low amino acids don't just *cause* depression. When depression sets in, levels of amino acids drop even further—and a more severe period of depression may be triggered by those lower levels.

Physical and mental fatigue—common symptoms of depression—also deplete amino acid levels.

Amino acid levels in the blood (and in platelets, blood components that play a role in clotting) may determine whether or not a person is responsive to antidepressant medications for major depression. The lower the levels, the less responsive.

Are you getting the idea that normal amino acid levels are a *must* for generating neurotransmitters—and preventing and treating depression? I hope so!

What Happens When You Block Tryptophan Production in the Body?

Animal and human studies on "acute tryptophan depletion" (ATD) show that when this serotonin-creating amino acid is missing, the brain suffers. And behavior with it.

In an ATD study, the subjects of the study are given a drink with all amino acids *except* tryptophan, which causes tryptophan levels in the brain to plummet. Serotonin production follows, dropping dramatically. And the change in behavior is like Dr. Jekyll changing into Mr. Hyde.

Learning and memory are impaired. Subjects are more impulsive and aggressive. Various brain functions go into low gear. Instability rather than balance is the norm.

My clinical experience matches these studies. When tryptophan and other amino acids are low, my patients are more likely to suffer from depression, mood swings, anxiety, impulsiveness, irritability and agitation, and aggression.

Do You Have a Deficiency?

Getting amino acids in your diet isn't that difficult. They're found in protein-rich foods like meat, eggs, and beans, and most people get enough protein in their ordinary diet. But even if you get plenty of protein, you can still end up with low blood levels of amino acids.

I started testing for "fasting plasma amino acids" more than thirty years ago—and I found the results mind-boggling! I expected blood levels of amino acids to reflect what the patient had eaten the night before: if it was a high-carb meal, numbers should be low; if it was a steak, numbers should be high. But after thousands of tests, I was surprised to learn that levels of fasting plasma amino acids had very little to do with dietary intake. Patients with severely restricted diets—like people with anorexia nervosa—would have normal levels. People who ate protein three times a day might have very low levels. Eventually, I figured out that protein *intake* didn't determine levels of amino acids; it was protein *absorption* that made all the difference.

For one thing, the stomach has to contain sufficient stomach acid and digestive enzymes like pepsin to start the process of protein digestion. This is a complex process, and a lot can go wrong—and often does.

You can have too little stomach acid, a common problem. (A 40 percent reduction in stomach acid typically occurs between your teens and thirties, with an additional 50 percent decline by the time you're seventy.) You might also be taking antacids, which work by blocking the production of stomach acid.

Protein digestion and absorption is also hampered by low levels of digestive enzymes, compounds that help with the efficient and complete breakdown of food into its digestible parts, like turning protein into amino acids. Some signs that you may be low in digestive enzymes are feeling full soon after starting to eat, abdominal pain after meals, bloating and gas, and diarrhea.

The physiological demand for normal levels of stomach acid and digestive enzymes illustrates what I call the "Laws of Essential Nutrition," which expand the familiar saying, "You are what you eat." The three laws:

1. You are what you eat.

2. You are what you *don't* eat.

3. You are what you can digest/absorb.

Another factor in protein digestion: the "fight-or-flight" stress response, which reduces the blood flow aiding protein digestion, sending it instead to the muscles. Chronic stress leads to chronic indigestion—and poor absorption of amino acids.

Bottom line: If you can't break down protein effectively into individual amino acids, it doesn't matter how much protein you consume. Increasing protein in your diet is *not* the answer.

What is?

Providing a protein source that is predigested.

Free-Form Amino Acids: Highly Absorbable, Highly Effective

When you consume free-form amino acids, *no* digestion is required—the amino acids are absorbed directly into the bloodstream. This makes them easily available to every structure and function in the body—including the brain, and its formation and regulation of neurotransmitters.

Since people struggling with depression (and anxiety, and fatigue) often suffer from an underlying amino acid deficiency, providing the raw materials they need can have a rapid and dramatic result on their health.

Bottom line: For thousands of patients, supplementation with free-form amino acids has been one of the most consistent and effective approaches to improve and restore mood.

And the changes can be quick—often within two weeks. Mood is elevated. Energy increases. Irritability evaporates. The depressed person often describes a "night-and-day" difference.

(Other benefits of free-form amino acids can include enhanced athlete training, improved strength, faster recovery after exercise, and a stronger immune system.)

Recommended product

There are many amino acid products on the market. I recommend Amino Acid Replete, from Pure Encapsulations, which is one of the few free-form amino acid products on the market that contains a broad spectrum of amino acids in their proper, biological ratios—including tryptophan, which is the amino acid that's absolutely necessary as a precursor to serotonin. Most amino acids formulas *don't* include tryptophan—and they could actually make you feel worse.

Suggested Dose: Take one scoop (4 grams, or g) twice daily, in a glass of water or juice *between* meals. Don't mix with a protein-rich liquid, like yogurt or milk, which will decrease absorption.

Supplement with digestive enzymes and hydrochloric acid (HCl)

Along with free-form amino acids, I recommend taking two other compounds that ensure efficient protein digestion: digestive enzymes, which help break down protein into a digestible form; and HCl, the equivalent of stomach acid. You can find both of these compounds in the product Digestive Enzymes Ultra with Betaine HCl, from Pure Encapsulations. Take one capsule with every meal: breakfast, lunch, and dinner. You can find similar digestive enzyme/HCl formulations from other companies. Just make sure they contain Betaine HCl—the lack of this ingredient is the number one reason people with low levels of amino acids don't experience improvement.

Don't worry about drug/supplement interactions: you can safely take a digestive enzyme/HCl supplement with an antidepressant medication.

Boosting serotonin and dopamine

In my practice, I often recommend a serotonin- and dopamine-boosting supplement that I formulated: NeuroPure, from Pure Encapsulations. This supplement supplies 5-HTP to boost serotonin, and DL-phenylalanine to boost dopamine. (Using this product is a smart exception to my rule that you shouldn't take individual amino acids without your doctor's approval and supervision because it's formulated for a balanced effect.) NeuroPure also provides several other nutritional cofactors for neurotransmitters that you'll read about in the upcoming chapters, like zinc, vitamin B6, and folate. Plus, it delivers curcumin and quercetin, plant compounds that reduce neuroinflammation, another factor in depression. (I also find this supplement effective in treating binge eating disorder.)

However, if you're taking an antidepressant, this supplement is not for you—the medication and the supplement together could produce too much serotonin.

But if you're not currently taking an antidepressant and want relief from depression, or you want to prevent depression or a relapse, this supplement is ideal for you.

The two basic amino acid protocols I'm suggesting in this chapter look like this:

If you're depressed and not on an antidepressant, take 1) free-form amino acids; 2) NeuroPure; and 3) a supplement containing digestive enzymes and HCl.

If you're depressed and on an antidepressant, take 1) a supplement of free-form amino acids; and 2) a supplement containing digestive enzymes and HCl. Do not take NeuroPure.

I consider NeuroPure to be a *nutraceutical*—a supplement that delivers high doses of specific nutrients, producing a pharmacological effect.

Should You Test First?

Should your doctor test for amino acids? Throughout this book, I recommended first *testing* for specific biochemical imbalances that cause or contribute to depression and then *treating* if an imbalance is detected. *Test, don't guess* is one of my therapeutic mantras (in addition to *first test, then treat*).

Amino acid testing provides valuable information, possibly revealing low levels of amino acids, a sure indicator that you should be taking free-form amino acids, and a digestive enzyme/HCl supplement. Plasma or urinary amino acid tests are available. It's important to get a *fasting* level for the most accurate results—so take the test first thing in the morning, before eating.

But even *without* testing, supplementing with free-form amino acids is often an effective (and very safe) strategy for reversing depression. (It also works for managing withdrawal from antidepressants, as you'll learn in Chapter 17.) In fact, I *always* give a free-form amino acid supplement to a depressed patient—regardless of testing—because of the consistent success and safety of this powerful therapy. Likewise, you should feel free to take this powerful supplement without talking to your doctor first. (That's why it's part of the Essential Functional Psychiatry Plan, which I present in Chapter 2—the supplements you can start taking *now*, without testing.)

It's also important to note that I don't rush to treat low levels of *specific* amino acids. I have found that correcting specific deficiencies of amino acids rarely makes a difference in the patient's experience. Giving the thirteen free-form amino acids that are found in Amino Replete corrects deficiencies in phenylalanine, tyrosine, and tryptophan, the amino acids that play the most significant role in forming the neurotransmitters that fight depression. Giving NeuroPure provides 5-HTP and phenylalanine, raising levels of serotonin and dopamine. Work with your doctor to see what's best for *you*. Individualized medicine—functional medicine—is the key to real prevention and treatment.

Free-Form Amino Acids

Use this practical, step-by-step summary to implement the therapeutic actions discussed in this chapter.

Step #1: Take a free-form amino acid supplement. I recommend the product Amino Replete, from Pure Encapsulations.

> **Suggested dose:** Take one scoop (4 g) twice daily, in a glass of water or juice between meals. Don't mix with a protein-rich liquid, like yogurt or milk, which will decrease absorption.

Step #2: Take a supplement combining digestive enzymes and HCl, with breakfast, lunch, and dinner. I recommend Digestive Enzymes Ultra, with Betaine HCl, from Pure Encapsulations.

> **Suggested dose:** Take one to two capsules at the start of every meal.

Step #3: Consider taking the serotonin and dopamine booster NeuroPure, from Pure Encapsulations, if you are currently *not* taking antidepressants.

> **Suggested dose:** Two capsules per day, one before breakfast and one before dinner. After one month, increase to four capsules daily, two before breakfast and two before dinner.

Step #4: If you have excessive rumination—repetitive, near-constant thinking about problems and negative events, in the past, present, or imagined future—consider taking 5-HTP, a serotonin precursor, if you are currently *not* taking antidepressants.

> **Suggested dose:** 50 to 200 mg, in two divided doses (breakfast and dinner). Start low and increase gradually—5-HTP can cause stomach upset, gas, and cramping.

> **Contraindications:** Never take 5-HTP if you are also taking antidepressants. And if you have a history of bipolar illness, you can

become anxious and agitated on the supplement, even to the point of suicidality.

Step #5: Talk to your doctor about possible testing for amino acid levels—the fasting plasma test is preferable. A pattern of low levels confirms your need for free-form amino acids. Testing, however, is not necessary to follow Steps #1 through #4.

CHAPTER 5

Vitamin D

D Is for Depression-Fighter

> Vitamin D is a must for normal levels
> of serotonin. But depression-causing
> deficiencies are common.

What a difference a few decades make.

Thirty years ago, cell phones were for talking only. And thirty years ago, vitamin D was considered a one-dimensional nutrient—good for calcium absorption and strong bones, but not much else.

Now, cell phones are indispensable for nearly every dimension of our lives. Now, scientists understand that vitamin D is indispensable to health and healing—a must not only for building bones, but also for a wide range of biochemical actions and health effects.

What happened in those thirty years?

Scientists discovered vitamin D receptors in cells throughout the body—providing a crucial clue that the nutrient is active in more than just the skeletal system.

Scientists also discovered more than one thousand brain-related genes that contain "vitamin D response elements." In other words, it takes vitamin D to activate those genes—genes responsible for maintaining the health of brain cells.

Plus, research has revealed the specific actions of vitamin D in many systems and organs:

In the endocrine glands, which generate hormones, the chemical messengers tasked with regulating all of the functions of the body.

In the liver, which purifies the body of toxins.

In the skin, which connects us with, and protects us from, the outside world.

In the immune system, which repels foreign invaders like bacteria and viruses.

In the digestive system, which assimilates food.

In the heart, which pumps life-giving blood through the body.

In the brain, which allows us to think, feel, and act.

And when the brain is imbalanced because of a lack of vitamin D, depression is far more likely.

But before we examine the role of vitamin D in depression, let's look more closely at the nutrient itself—what it is, and how it works.

Vitamin D 101

There are a lot of odd facts about vitamin D.

For starters, it's not exactly a vitamin (although everyone calls it that, and so we will, too, throughout this chapter). It's a *prohormone*, a substance the body converts into a hormone.

Another oddity: The main source of vitamin D isn't food. Only a few foods are naturally rich in vitamin D, like fatty fish (salmon, tuna, sardines, mackerel), cod liver oil, eggs (the yolks), beef liver, mushrooms, and Swiss cheese. (Although a lot of foods, like milk, yogurt, orange juice, and breakfast cereals, are fortified with the vitamin.)

But Mother Nature didn't leave your vitamin D intake up to chance, hoping you'll have a tuna mushroom omelet for breakfast. Instead of food, the body uses *sunlight* to supply vitamin D. In fact, sunlight typically accounts for 90 percent of the vitamin D in the body.

The process: When ultraviolet B (UVB) radiation hits the skin, it converts a cholesterol precursor (7-dehydrocholesterol) into the compound cholecalciferol.

Next, enzymes in the liver and kidney convert cholecalciferol to calcitriol (1,25-dihydroxycholecalciferol), the biologically active form of vitamin D, also known as D3. (The stored form of vitamin D—ergocalciferol—is vitamin D2.)

And D3 acts in a hormone-like fashion, as it binds to vitamin D receptors on cells. Its tasks include:

- regulating the amount of calcium and phosphorous in cells;

- making sure bone grows and is repaired;

- regulating cellular growth and division (making the vitamin a powerful foe of cancer);

- easing inflammation, the cause of many chronic diseases;

- strengthening the immune system, by boosting the activity of several types of white blood cells;

- fortifying the stress-protecting adrenal glands; and

- of great import to anybody with depression, increasing the production of the brain-regulating neurotransmitters serotonin, dopamine, and norepinephrine.

Vitamin D for Better Health

Given the breadth of its actions, it's no surprise that having too little vitamin D on board is linked to many health problems. For example, it helps prevent or treat:

Cancer, by regulating cell growth and decreasing the risk that cells become malignant.

High blood pressure, by managing the production of renin, a hormone that controls *vasodilation*, the narrowing and widening of arteries.

Frailty and falls in the elderly, by helping maintain muscle strength.

Autoimmune diseases, by enhancing the infection-fighting power of immune cells.

Type 2 diabetes, by regulating the metabolism of glucose (blood sugar), and maintaining insulin sensitivity, the ability of the hormone insulin to usher glucose out of the bloodstream and into cells.

Subpar Studies

Surprisingly, the results of clinical studies using vitamin D supplementation to prevent or reverse these conditions have been mixed. That's because the people who benefit the most from vitamin D supplements are those who have low blood levels of vitamin D—and studies rarely make a distinction between participants with normal and subpar levels of vitamin D. Sometimes vitamin D levels are *never* measured at any time during a study on vitamin D!

In other words, a person with healthy vitamin D levels who enrolls in a trial of vitamin D supplementation is unlikely to experience health benefits from the intervention—while a person who starts the trial with low levels will probably benefit.

I bring up this problem in studies and results because the therapeutic value of vitamin D is often dismissed by health professionals who look at the scientific literature and see mixed results.

But in my clinical practice—my actual day-to-day experience with thousands of patients over the last several decades—I have seen consistent, positive results in the power of vitamin D to help overcome depression. That's because I first *test* for low vitamin D levels, and then *treat* when levels are low.

(It's also important to note that many studies *do* show efficacy for vitamin D, with the COVID-19 pandemic providing yet another scientific demonstration of the power of the vitamin. Researchers at the University of Chicago showed that people with vitamin D deficiency were 77 percent more likely to be infected with COVID-19.[1] A French study of seventy-seven elderly patients hospitalized with COVID-19 found that those who took vitamin D supplements regularly during the year before the COVID-19 diagnosis were less likely to have severe disease and more likely to survive compared to people who didn't take vitamin D.[2] And in a study in the *Journal of Clinical Endocrinology & Metabolism*, COVID-19 patients with low vitamin D had a higher risk of intensive care unit admission and death than those with normal levels.[3] When it comes to COVID-19, getting enough vitamin D is essential.

Vitamin D and Your Mind

The *D* in vitamin D could stand for *Depression-fighter*. Here's why.

Vitamin D acts in regions of the brain that play a role in the development of depression, including the prefrontal cortex, hippocampus, cingulate gyrus, thalamus, hypothalamus, and substantia nigra.

Vitamin D receptors are found in both neurons and *glial cells*, the specialized brain cells that support neurons by providing nutrition and insulation.

Vitamin D may promote the release of *neurotrophins*, a family of proteins that protects neurons and stimulates their growth.

But most importantly, sufficient levels of vitamin D in the brain activate enzymes involved in the synthesis of three neurotransmitters, chemicals that transmit messages from neuron to neuron.

Serotonin. Vitamin D increases the production of *serotonin*, the "feel-good" neurotransmitter that regulates mood, sleep, appetite, and pain—all of which are commonly dysregulated in depression.

Dopamine. Vitamin D increases the production of *dopamine*, the neurotransmitter that provides a sense of accomplishment and feelings of pleasure—feelings that are sorely lacking in depression.

Norepinephrine. Vitamin D increases the production of *norepinephrine*, the neurotransmitter that regulates the "fight-or-flight" response—and therefore regulates whether you feel stressed or not. Norepinephrine also regulates attention and focus, and mood—with low levels linked to depression.

Vitamin D and Serotonin

Let's double back for a moment and take a look at vitamin D and serotonin.

Vitamin D regulates the production of serotonin—simply put, less vitamin D translates to less serotonin. The process works like this.

The amino acid tryptophan is processed by an enzyme called *tryptophan hydrolase* (TPH), which determines how slow or fast serotonin is manufactured. There are two forms of TPH: TPH1, found mainly in the gut; and TPH2, found mainly in the brain. Vitamin D is critical for the functioning of both TPH enzymes—making vitamin D a must for serotonin production in the brain.

Little wonder, then, that in a study that reviewed fifteen other studies on vitamin D and depression (a so-called "meta-analysis"), the researchers found that the effect of vitamin D supplements on depression "was comparable to that of anti-depressant medication."[4]

In other words, supplementing with vitamin D worked just as well as antidepressants!

Strong Studies on Vitamin D and Depression

The biochemical connection between neurotransmitters and vitamin D helps explain the results of many scientific studies linking low levels of vitamin D and depression. For example:

More vitamin D, less depression. In a study of more than eighty-one thousand postmenopausal women, those with the lowest levels of vitamin D had the greatest risk for depressive symptoms.[5] In another study, of more than three thousand European men, low levels of vitamin D were linked to depression.[6] And Australian researchers found a similar link between low D and depression in young men.[7]

Effective treatment. Depression is common in people with type 2 diabetes—the disease doubles the risk of depression, and an estimated one in three people with diabetes are depressed.

In one study on diabetes and depression, researchers looked at sixty-eight people with both health problems, dividing them into two groups. One group took 4,000 international units (IU) of vitamin D daily; the other group took a placebo.

After three months, blood levels of vitamin D in the supplemented group had doubled—and their scores on the Beck Depression Inventory (which measures symptoms like sadness, guilt, loss of interest in activities, and fatigue) decreased by about 30 percent. The depressive symptoms in the placebo group decreased only a little.

The researchers also note that the vitamin D group had several positive changes in the metabolic profile of diabetes: lower A1c (a measure of long-term blood sugar control); lower insulin (high levels of insulin are a feature of type 2 diabetes); and lower triglycerides (a heart-hurting blood fat).

"Supplementation of vitamin D in type 2 diabetes patients may protect these patients against the onset of major depressive disorders, with noticeable favorable effects on measures of metabolic profiles," wrote the researchers in *Diabetes & Metabolic Syndrome: Clinical Research & Reviews.*[8]

Depressed before, not depressed now. In a four-year study involving more than twelve thousand patients, people with a prior history of depression who had the highest blood levels of vitamin D were 10 percent less likely to be currently suffering from depression than those with lower levels.[9]

Saying no to negative emotions. Researchers from Taiwan analyzed the results of twenty-five studies with more than seven thousand participants—and found that supplementing with vitamin D can "reduce negative emotions" in people with major depression.[10]

In another study, from Australian researchers, healthy people were given either 800 IU of vitamin D, 400 IU of vitamin D, or no vitamin D during five days of winter. Those taking the vitamin had "significantly enhanced positive affect" (more positive emotions) and a "reduction in negative affect" (fewer negative emotions).[11]

Lower risk of suicide. In a Korean study of more than 150,000 people, vitamin D deficiency was linked with a 14 percent increased risk of suicide.[12]

And in a study of ninety-one adolescents—some who were depressed and had attempted suicide; some who were depressed but had not attempted suicide; and some who were healthy—58 percent of those who had attempted suicide were deficient in vitamin D.[13] In a similar study, published in the *Annals of Clinical Psychiatry*, researchers found that adolescents who had attempted suicide had an average level of vitamin D that was 37 percent lower than those who had not attempted suicide.[14]

Low D = high risk. A study from Dutch researchers, published in the medical journal *Molecular Psychiatry*, sums up the irrefutable connection between vitamin D and depression.

The researchers looked at 2,386 people: people who were currently depressed; people who were in remission from depression; and people who had never been depressed.

Overall, one-third of the study participants had deficient or insufficient blood levels of vitamin D. But the lowest levels were found in people who were currently depressed, particularly those with the most severe symptoms. In fact, the lower the level, the more severe the symptoms.

Low levels of vitamin D might "represent an underlying biological vulnerability for depression," wrote the researchers, suggesting that the vitamin could be "part of preventive or treatment interventions for depression."[15]

Bottom line: If you're depressed, vitamin D is an "intervention" you should consider very seriously!

Are You Deficient in Vitamin D?

It's pretty likely the answer is yes.

In the United States, up to 77 percent of adults and 67 percent of children are deficient in the vitamin. Why?

As I said earlier, few foods contain vitamin D.

Additionally, current medical advice says to always put sunscreen on before going outdoors—and sunscreen blocks the formation of vitamin D in the skin.

According to Michael Holick, MD, PhD, director of the Vitamin D, Skin and Bone Research Laboratory at Boston University Medical Center, you're at particular risk for low blood levels of vitamin D if you're:

Over sixty-five, because older skin makes less vitamin D. Fifty to 75 percent of seniors are deficient.

Overweight, because a high percentage of this fat-soluble vitamin gets deposited in your fat cells instead of circulating in your blood.

Finally Hopeful Success Story

PATIENT: Jayden

TREATMENT FOR: Severe depression

Jayden's parents came to me asking for help for their son, a seventeen-year-old African American struggling with severe depression.

Up until a year before, Jayden, now a senior in high school, had been getting decent grades, had an active social life, and played basketball and tennis for his school. But over the past year, he'd developed severe symptoms of depression, including a sense of being overwhelmed, and he'd dropped out of sports. He struggled to attend class, and his grades plummeted. His teachers proposed holding him back a year, delaying his graduation from high school.

My initial testing revealed severe vitamin D deficiency—a blood level of 6 nanograms per milliliter (ng/mL). Anything under 30 ng/mL is deficient; Jayden had next to no vitamin D in his blood.

I started treating him with 5,000 IU of vitamin D daily. After two months, Jayden's vitamin D levels had risen into the normal range—and his symptoms of depression diminished to the point where he reengaged with his schoolwork and other high school activities, including sports. His parents and teachers—and best of all, Jayden himself—were thrilled with his progress. And his teachers were no longer talking about holding him back—he was on track to graduate with his friends.

It's obvious that Jayden's depression has a single, treatable cause: vitamin D deficiency.

African American, Hispanic, or a person of color, because darker skin blocks vitamin D production.

Not a resident of the South or Southwest, where sun exposure is optimal.

Diagnosed with osteoporosis, a problem caused and worsened by low levels of vitamin D.

But the best way to know if you're deficient is a blood test.

Your doctor should test for 25-hydroxy vitamin D, which is the form of vitamin D the body uses for storage.

The test results are typically reported in ng/mL. Here's what your results mean:

- < 20, severe deficiency

- 20–30, insufficiency

- 30–40, low-normal

- 40–60, optimal

And if you're deficient, here's what to do.

Restoring Optimal Levels of Vitamin D

The best, simplest, and most dependable method for remedying a deficiency or insufficiency is taking a supplement of vitamin D3.

I recommend 2,000 to 10,000 IU daily, depending on the test results. In other words, the ideal scenario is: Test *first* and *then* start supplementation.

A possible framework to discuss with your doctor: 2,000 IU daily for optimal; 3,000 to 4,000 for low-normal; 4,000 to 6,000 for insufficiency; and 6,000 to 10,000 for severe deficiency.

I also recommend testing twice a year (at least), to monitor any possible fluctuations in vitamin D levels—and to confirm that levels remain in the optimal range.

Biochemical Individuality Makes Testing a Must

Biochemical individuality—unique differences in genetics, metabolism, and nutritional needs—plays a role in vitamin D levels and the need for supplementation.

A Swedish study of same-sex twins found that genetic factors caused 25 percent of the variations in vitamin D levels, independent of season (your skin makes more vitamin D during the summer months).

And during the summer, genes accounted for 50 percent of the variations. In other words, even if you're getting a lot of sunlight, you may not be making vitamin D—because of your genetic makeup.[16]

That's why testing is an absolute must—no matter how much vitamin D you're getting from sunlight and diet.

In patients with depression, I recommend continuing supplementation indefinitely, to keep levels optimal, supplementing at 2,000 IU daily.

That's because depressed patients tend to become deficient six months to a year after stopping supplementation, and we want to prevent that!

I'd like to add that a few people *do* maintain optimal levels of vitamin D, through sun exposure and eating plenty of D-rich and D-fortified foods.

In those folks, there's no need to supplement.

In terms of getting vitamin D from sunlight: levels are so variable by time of day, season of the year, latitude, and skin pigmentation, that no single recommendation can assure adequate levels. But here's a good rule of thumb, from Dr. Holick:

Spend ten to fifteen minutes, three to four times a week in the sun, without sunscreen on your arms, legs, and hands. After fifteen minutes, apply sunscreen to these areas. Never sun to the point of burning. Always protect your face with a sunscreen or hat.

Vitamin D also needs help from some other nutrients to do its job.

The first is the mineral magnesium, without which vitamin D can't convert into its active form. I recommend a minimum of 240 mg daily of magnesium glycinate: 120 mg, twice a day, at breakfast and before bed. (Magnesium relaxes muscles and nerves, and aids sleep.)

The second is vitamin K2, which is now routinely added to many vitamin D supplements. Vitamin D3 helps the body absorb and use calcium—taking K2 with D3 helps to ensure the calcium is absorbed by your bones (where it's needed) rather than accumulating in your arteries (where it's not).

STEP-BY-STEP ACTION PLAN FOR

Vitamin D

Use this practical, step-by-step summary to implement the therapeutic actions discussed in this chapter.

Step #1: It's always best to get tested for blood vitamin D levels—because it's impossible to determine the supplemental dosage you need without a test for blood levels.

Step #2: Retest after three months of supplementation, adjusting dose as needed. For subsequent years, test twice yearly, adjusting dose as needed.

Step #3: Based on the results of the test, take between 2,000 and 10,000 IU per day. The general guidelines are:

- < 20, severe deficiency: 10,000 IU daily for three months, at which point test again and adjust the dose.

- 20–30, insufficiency: 5,000 IU daily

- 30–40, low-normal: 2,000 IU daily

- 40–60, optimal: No need for supplementation

Step #4: Take a supplement that includes vitamin K2, which ensures that the calcium absorbed because of vitamin D ends up in your bones rather than your arteries.

Step #5: Take magnesium, an important cofactor for vitamin D to create serotonin. Dose: 120 mg of magnesium glycinate, twice a day, at breakfast and bedtime.

Step #6: Help maintain sufficient exposure to sunlight to generate vitamin D levels. A good strategy: Spend ten to fifteen minutes, three to four times a week in the sun, without sunscreen on your arms, legs, and hands. After fifteen minutes, apply sunscreen to these areas. Never sun to the point of burning. Always protect your face with a sunscreen or hat.

Step #7: Maintain dietary intake of vitamin D, with two to three servings per week of fatty fish like salmon, tuna, sardines, and anchovies, and D-fortified foods like milk, orange juice, and breakfast cereal.

Step #8: If you have suffered from depression at any time during your life—and even if you're currently in remission—continue supplementing with 2,000 IU of vitamin D3 daily (with vitamin K2) to ensure you maintain optimal blood levels.

CHAPTER 6

B Vitamins

Building Blocks of a Better Brain

> These key nutrients repair your depleted brain.

A word with a *B* attached to it usually indicates something is second-rate. "B-list" celebrities are eager to make the A-list. Players on the "B-team" aren't as talented as the starters. "B-movies" have low budgets. "B-grade" meat is loaded with gristle.

But there's nothing second-rate about the vitamins labeled *B*. Without them, there's no way you're going to have first-rate health—or a first-rate brain. They got their *B* label only because they were discovered after vitamin A (and before vitamin C).

In the early twentieth century, scientists thought all the Bs were a single vitamin. Over time, they realized that each B vitamin—from vitamin B1 (thiamine) to vitamin B12 (cobalamin)—is distinct. And distinctly important to health.

Among their many key functions, B vitamins: make and repair DNA; oversee the growth and development of cells; help convert food into energy; and produce red blood cells (RBCs). In other words, B vitamins are definitely not on the biochemical B-list!

And as you'll discover in this chapter, the *B* in B vitamins could stand for *brain*. They play key roles in brain health, feeding neurons, helping produce neurotransmitters—and fighting depression.

Let's take a look at the most important Bs for optimal brain health and mental well-being—starting with vitamin B12.

Vitamin B12:
Deficiency and Depression

B12 is as important to your body as tires are to a car. B12 is a must in the creation of DNA, the cellular instruction manual that guides all the activities of body and mind. It's crucial in the formation of red blood cells, which carry oxygen to every cell, tissue, and organ in the body. It's a key step in regulating *methylation pathways,* basic biological processes that sustain cells. B12 also works with folate and B6 to produce serotonin and dopamine, two neurotransmitters that are part of the foundation of positive mood.

In fact, B12—sometimes called the "feel-good" vitamin—is downright brainy. It's central to the health of every nerve cell (neuron) in the body—and therefore the health of the brain, the spinal cord, and all the nerves that extend from the spinal cord, like branches from the trunk of a tree.

B12 stimulates the production of *neuronal growth factors*, proteins that are critical to the growth, development, and survival of neurons. Low levels of these growth factors—like brain-derived neurotrophic factor (BDNF)—are linked to depression, anxiety, Alzheimer's disease, Parkinson's disease, and schizophrenia.

B12 also protects *myelin*, the fatty coating that shields nerves from damage.

So it's not surprising that low blood levels of B12 have been linked to many mental health problems, including depression, mania, anxiety, paranoia, memory loss, behavioral changes, and psychosis.

And by linked, I mean *strongly* linked. For example, in a study of patients admitted to a psychiatric hospital, one in three had a deficiency of B12.

But the link with depression is even stronger. Studies show that up to 70 percent of depressed patients have a B12 deficiency! Let's look at some of the research.

Low B12, high risk of depression. In a study by Dutch researchers of nearly four thousand seniors, low levels of vitamin B12 were directly linked to depressive symptoms and depressive disorders. "Vitamin B12 may be causally related to depression," wrote the researchers in the *American Journal of Psychiatry*. In other words, low levels of B12 might *cause* depression![1]

Less sadness with B12. When Finnish researchers studied people with major depressive disorder (MDD), they found those who were treated with B12 for six months had fewer and less severe depressive symptoms, like sadness, pessimism, guilt, insomnia, and apathy.[2]

And those are just a few of the *hundreds* of studies on B12 and depression.

As I was starting this book, I searched the medical database of the National Institutes of Health, using the keywords "depression" and "B12"—and turned up several recent studies on depression and B12. They included these findings:

Adolescents with depression were more likely to have lower levels of B12, according to a study in *Neuropsychiatric Disease and Treatment*.[3]

In a study of nearly eighteen thousand people, **those with the highest intake of B12 were 35 percent less likely to be depressed**. Researchers also linked high levels of vitamin B1 and B6 to lower risk of depression. The results were published in the *International Journal of Vitamin and Nutrition Research*.[4]

Supplementing the diet with vitamin B12 "significantly decreased depression," either as a stand-alone therapy or by improving the response to medication, according to a study in *Nutritional Neuroscience*.[5]

Researchers from the University of Pennsylvania looked at thirty-two studies on diet and depression—and found **a direct link between higher dietary intake of vitamin B12 and fewer depressive symptoms**. The results were published in *Health Promotion Perspectives*.[6]

Postpartum depression (PD) is much less likely in women with the highest levels of vitamin B12, according to Spanish researchers in the *Journal of Reproductive and Infant Psychology*.[7]

Depressed people over sixty who attempt suicide have lower levels of vitamin B12 than depressed people who don't attempt suicide, according to a study published in *BMC Geriatrics*.[8]

In a review of fifty-six studies involving nearly thirty-eight thousand children and adolescents, **those with the highest levels of vitamin B12 were 21 percent less likely to be depressed** (and 17 percent less likely

Finally Hopeful Success Story

PATIENT: Sally

TREATMENT FOR: Depression, anxiety, and emotional eating

Sally was a thirty-three-year-old with depression, anxiety, and emotional eating. She told me she "always" felt sad and irritable, and experienced one to two panic attacks every week. She ate when she felt stressed, and struggled with her weight. Her primary care physician had prescribed an antidepressant, but Sally said she preferred to go the "natural route"—and so had scheduled a visit with me.

Testing showed that Sally's vitamin B12 was quite low, at 273 picograms per milliliter (pg/mL). She also had low levels of ferritin (a sign of iron deficiency) and low levels of multiple amino acids.

I started her on 2,000 micrograms (mcg) per day of vitamin B12 (methylcobalamin), using a sublingual pill (applied under the tongue) for faster, better absorption. She also took a daily iron supplement, free-form amino acids, and magnesium glycinate. I counseled her to increase her intake of dietary protein and vegetables, and to reduce refined carbohydrates.

After two months of feeling better, Sally was significantly improved. She told me she felt less depressed and anxious, she hardly ever had a panic attack anymore, and her moods were more stable. She didn't feel compelled to eat when she was stressed and was slowly but surely losing weight. She also said she had more energy and better concentration.

And sure enough, when I tested her B12 levels, they were at 536 pg/mL—normalized. Her iron also increased, as did her amino acid levels. Once again, the approach of Functional Psychiatry—*first test, then treat*—showed its efficacy. And Sally was a much happier person as a result.

to have behavioral problems). The research appeared in *Psychopharma-cology and Neuroscience.*[9]

Over decades of clinical practice, I've seen B12 work to relieve the symptoms of thousands of depressed patients. It's likely it can help you, too.

Testing for B12:
Clearing up the Confusion

Every person who is depressed should have their B12 levels checked, without exception. The link between B12 and depression is that straight-forward.

Unfortunately, interpreting B12 testing is not straightforward. There are many misconceptions among medical experts as to what B12 levels mean, and what should be done about them.

I'd go so far as to say that the confusion about B12 testing and sup-plementation is one of the greatest tragedies in modern medicine. I'm not exaggerating. This safe, biologically essential vitamin confers a mul-titude of therapeutic benefits to patients. It can restore energy, clear up brain fog, reduce the risk of heart disease, balance metabolism, and de-feat depression (not to mention a range of other mental health prob-lems). But low levels are routinely overlooked by conventional doctors.

Three misconceptions

There are three main misconceptions around B12 testing:

Misconception #1: Serum levels are an accurate and effective way to measure B12 status. Serum is the liquid portion of blood, and doesn't contain any blood cells. But what a serum test does *not* reveal is how much B12 is circulating and available in the cerebrospinal fluid of the brain—which is where B12 is actually utilized for mental health. So even a normal or high level of serum B12 does *not* tell us how much B12 is reaching the neurons in the brain.

Clinically, I've seen many cases where serum B12 is normal—but patients had a marked deficiency. This is particularly common in people with cancer, liver disease, or kidney disease. And that's a lot of people: 40 percent of Americans will develop cancer at some time in their lives; one hundred million Americans have fatty liver disease; and 15 percent of adults have chronic kidney disease.

Misconception #2: Vitamin B12 deficiency always causes *macrocytic anemia*. In this condition, low levels of B12 (or folate) cause larger-than-normal blood cells that do a subpar job of carrying oxygen to the cells. Possible symptoms include fatigue, weakness, and shortness of breath, along with neurological problems like numbness and tingling in the hands and feet. But doctors assume if there is no macrocytic anemia, the B12 level is normal. But that is *not* the case. You can have B12 deficiency without macrocytic anemia—and many people do.

Misconception #3: B12 deficiency is uncommon—and only becomes common as people age. B12 deficiency is very common—with one study showing that 40 percent of Americans have low levels, and 20 percent of seniors have severe vitamin B12 deficiency (because of a declining ability to absorb the vitamin). Vegetarians and vegans are also at risk: B12 is created by bacteria and other single-cell organisms in the bodies of animals, and is found mainly in animal foods like meat, fish, poultry, eggs, and dairy products. In a study in the *American Journal of Clinical Nutrition*, researchers found low vitamin B12 levels in 77 percent of vegetarians and 92 percent of vegans.[10]

Why these misconceptions about B12 deficiency?

1. The way the body utilizes B12 is very individual.

2. Testing for B12 is challenging, with technical limitations.

What does "normal" really mean?

The concept of "biochemical individuality" tells us that no two people are exactly alike when it comes to nutritional needs—some need more of a nutrient; some need less. The concept also says that what happens to the body and mind when there is a nutritional deficiency is different in the case of each individual. Which means there is no "classic" picture of symptoms from a B12 deficiency. It's entirely possible for ten different people suffering from low B12 levels to have ten different sets of symptoms. Which in turn means that testing is *always* a must—it's the only way to determine if levels are low.

And testing itself presents its own challenges.

What is "normal"? (No one really knows!) B12 levels that are considered "normal" vary—from laboratory to laboratory! This variance is caused by the fact that "normal" is determined by statistical averages

Where Antidepressants Failed, B12 Worked

A paper in the journal *Psychiatry* describes two patients who were resistant to antidepressants—but not to B12.[11]

In one case, a forty-three-year-old man—with a history of insomnia that had developed into major depression—had been unsuccessfully treated with various combinations of Tofranil (imipramine), Prozac (fluoxetine), Anafranil (clomipramine), Remeron (mirtazapine), Lexapro (escitalopram), and Savella (milnacipran).

In the second case, a twenty-nine-year-old man had MDD for five years, and had taken Lexapro, Effexor (venlafaxine), and Tofranil. With no results.

The doctor found out that both men were vegetarians—and testing showed both had low B12 levels.

The forty-three-year-old was given 1,000 micrograms (mcg) per day of vitamin B12 in addition to his antidepressant medication—and his symptoms improved within three weeks. He continued to take B12 every day—and at a follow-up eighteen months later, his symptoms continued to be much improved.

The twenty-nine-year-old was also treated with 1,000 mcg per day of B12 along with his medication. His depression improved after four weeks.

derived from large groups of tested people. Normal in Boston might be very different from normal in Los Angeles. It just depends on the lab.

"Normal" may be deficient. Research shows that the "normal" parameters applied by most laboratories are far too broad, ranging from 200 to 1,100 pg/mL. Some labs say levels as low as 150 are normal. Four to five hundred is likely the more accurate measurement below which deficiency is a reality. In other words, a lab might tell you 200 is normal—but it's actually a deficiency. My clinical experience has shown that cases of depression where B12 is under 500 will usually respond to B12 supplementation.

"Normal" doesn't mean optimal. And even *if* a patient's levels are within the so-called normal range, that doesn't mean all is biologically well. The individual may need a lot more B12 to function normally. In my clinical experience, it's possible for one patient with a serum level of 340 to feel fine, while another patient with the exact same level is suffering from symptoms of B12 deficiency—including depression.

Two more biomarkers

I recommend looking at two other biomarkers, to create an accurate picture of B12 status.

Homocysteine. This amino acid is frequently elevated in cases of vitamin B12 (and folate) deficiency. High homocysteine has been linked to a range of neurological problems, including memory decline, poor judgment, Parkinson's disease, and Alzheimer's disease.

In fact, high homocysteine nearly *doubles* a person's risk of the brain atrophy that often precedes dementia. And Alzheimer's patients consistently have severely elevated levels of serum homocysteine. The link is so strong that some experts theorize excess homocysteine *causes* Alzheimer's disease—a perspective dubbed "the homocysteine hypothesis." In 2018, an international team of experts published a paper on the hypothesis, writing, "We . . . conclude that elevated plasma total homocysteine is a modifiable risk factor for the development of cognitive decline, dementia, and Alzheimer's disease in older persons." (High homocysteine doesn't only hurt the brain. It's also been linked to heart disease, stroke, and kidney disease.)[12]

If homocysteine levels are high, they can easily be reduced by supplementing the diet with B12, folate, and B6.

The "normal" range of homocysteine in the blood is between 5 and 15 micromoles per liter (μmol/L)—but I consider levels above 12 elevated.

Methylmalonic acid (MMA). This is a breakdown product (or metabolite) of amino acids. When it's high, B12 levels are likely to be low. Levels above 245 nanomoles per liter (nmol/L) mean you probably need more B12, or have an outright deficiency.

However, I have seen patients with low MMA *and* low B12. So I don't recommend MMA as the only means of assessing a person's B12 status. It's just a helpful addition to conventional testing.

Supplementing with Vitamin B12

The most natural way to raise the level of any nutrient in the body is by eating foods rich in that nutrient, and that goes for B12, which is found primarily in beef, fish, chicken, eggs, milk, cheese, and yogurt. But you could eat a steak a day and still not get enough B12 on board—because there are many factors that can get in the way of B12 absorption. For example:

Stomach acid. Sufficient amounts of stomach acid are a must for absorbing B12. But plenty of people have low levels of stomach acid—including the fifteen million Americans who regularly take an acid-blocking proton pump inhibitor (PPI) like Nexium, Prevacid, or Prilosec. Older people are also at risk: by the age of seventy, there's a 50 percent reduction in the secretion of stomach acid compared to the amount produced in our teens.

Intrinsic factor. The stomach lining doesn't only secrete stomach acid. It also secretes a protein called *intrinsic factor*—which binds to B12, ushering it out of the stomach and into the intestines, where the nutrient is absorbed by specialized cells called *enterocytes*. (This B12-specific failsafe mechanism gives you an idea of how crucial B12 is to the body's day-to-day health.) Like stomach acid, levels of intrinsic factor

Finally Hopeful Success Story

PATIENT: Alex, a sixty-year-old man
TREATED FOR: Severe depression, poor sleep

Alex—a contractor with a long history of severe depression—was struggling more than usual. For years, he had gotten by—even with a very stressful job—and managed to stay functional, taking 450 mg of Wellbutrin (bupropion XL) daily. But now he felt overwhelmed. His sleep was fitful. In the mornings, he struggled to get out of bed, delaying the start of his workday for hours. He felt guilt over his job performance. He felt tired all the time. And he felt hopeless. At that point, he called me.

After conducting a detailed physical and history, and listening to his story, I ordered laboratory tests.

Alex had low-normal B12, high homocysteine, and low vitamin D.

Based on those results, I proposed this Functional Psychiatry Treatment Plan to Alex:

- methylcobalamin (vitamin B12) injections, 1,000 mcg, two times per week, for one month;
- 5,000 IU of vitamin D;
- 2,000 mg of fish oil (omega-3); and
- 360 mg of magnesium glycinate, 120 mg in the morning, 240 mg in the evening.

decline with age. PPIs also block intrinsic factor. Autoimmune disease—which afflicts one out of every five Americans—cuts levels of intrinsic factor, too.

Fortunately, there's an easy way to bypass the stomach and virtually guarantee B12 levels are restored: *injections* of B12, which work quickly to restore normal levels. The best forms of injectable B12 are: *hydroxocobalamin*, which is a precursor to the active form of B12; and *methylcobalamin*, which is the active form of B12 that is used by the tissues of the body.

My reasoning:

Low vitamin B12 is often a part of the picture in depression. Supplementing with the nutrient can ease depression—and improve the performance of an antidepressant.

High levels of homocysteine are often caused by low levels of B12 and folate, and can contribute to depressive symptoms. Injections are the fastest way to restore B12 levels—and mood and energy quickly improve.

Low vitamin D is linked to depression, and supplementing with the nutrient improves depression.

Magnesium supports vitamin D, and aids restful sleep.

People with depression are often low in omega-3. I didn't test Alex for omega-3, but significant research links low levels of omega-3 to depression, and fish oil is a safe source of omega-3.

Alex agreed to the protocol, and I saw him two months later. His improvements were dramatic.

His sleep was deeper and more refreshing. His mood had improved, and he expressed hope for his future. He had more energy and was able to go back to work. Emotionally, he had reconnected with his wife and son. And all this had happened without any change in the stress of daily life—but targeted nutritional therapy optimized Alex's biochemistry, strengthening him in every way.

I recommend injections of 1,000 mcg, two times per week. Continue the injections monthly, if needed.

If you get injections, it's likely your B12 levels will become elevated—that is, they will rise significantly *above* the so-called "normal" range. That's not a problem—and definitely not a reason to stop treatment. The National Academy of Medicine (a nonprofit division of the esteemed National Academy of Sciences) has never established an upper limit of safety for doses of B12. In other words, they regard dosing with the vitamin as *very* safe. And they're right.

However, many people don't have the inclination, time, or funds to get injections. For them, oral supplementation is the best bet.

Vegetarians and Vegans Beware: You Need More B12!

Are vegetarians and vegans more likely to be depressed—because they're not getting enough vitamin B12, a nutrient that's found mainly in meat, poultry, fish, eggs, and dairy?

A study published in *Nutrition Reviews* in 2021 answers that question with a resounding yes.

The researchers analyzed the results of thirteen studies on vegan/vegetarian diets and mental health, involving nearly eighteen thousand people. The conclusion:

Vegans/vegetarians were *twice* as likely to be depressed!

These researchers didn't look at B12 levels in vegans/vegetarians, but plenty of others have. And the results show low B12 intake in vegans/vegetarians is very common. For example:

In a study involving sixty-five thousand people, the average B12 intake among meat eaters was 7.2 mcg, but only 0.4 mcg in vegans—180 times less!

And low intake inevitably leads to deficiency. A review of studies found that 60 percent of vegans and 40 percent of lacto-ovo vegetarians (a vegetarian diet that includes eggs and dairy) were deficient in B12. Other research has found that up to 90 percent of vegetarian adults are deficient.

Bottom line: If you're a vegetarian or vegan and you're depressed, you *must* take a B12 supplement. (It's a good idea even if you're not depressed!)[13]

For oral supplementation, I recommend PureMelt B12 Folate, from Pure Encapsulations. It delivers B12 in the form of methylcobalamin, the most biologically active form of the nutrient. The supplement also includes folate (which you'll read about in the next section of this chapter). And, most importantly, it's a "sublingual" form of the nutrient—a dissolvable pill placed under the tongue, where B12 can be absorbed easily and quickly. If you're eating meat and not absorbing B12—the exact situation with many of my depressed patients—then you *must* take a sublingual form of the vitamin. Take a daily dose of 2,000 mcg, twice per day.

There is one caution about taking B12 in the form of methylcobalamin: it can be stimulating, triggering agitation or worsening anxiety. If you have a history of anxiety, use hydroxocobalamin.

Folate (Vitamin B9)

When it comes to folate, the first thing to do is define our terms—because there are several forms of folate, and they work very differently in the body. The most commonly discussed forms are:

Folic acid. This is the synthetic form of the nutrient.

Folate. The natural form of the vitamin, found in foods like vegetables and legumes.

L-methylfolate (LMF). This is the biologically active form of the vitamin: It readily crosses the blood-brain barrier, the specialized cells that line the blood vessels of the brain, filtering out toxins.

Like B12, folate is a must for making DNA, and for the growth and development of cells. It also plays a role in translating DNA into RNA, which is then utilized by ribosomes, the structures in the cell that manufacture proteins. Working with B12, folate is key in methylation, particularly the methylation pathways that create serotonin, dopamine, and norepinephrine, the three neurotransmitters so essential for preventing and reversing depression. So it's not surprising that when folate levels are low, depression is more likely. (And they're frequently low, affecting an estimated 20 percent of Americans.)

There's plenty of scientific evidence demonstrating the link between low levels of folate and feeling low.

Low levels of folate, high risk of depression. In a recent study, low dietary intake and low blood levels of folate were linked to a higher risk of depression. "Clinicians may wish to consider folate supplementation for patients with depression," write the authors, in the *Journal of Psychiatric Research*.[14]

Double the risk of depression. In a study of more than 1,500 people aged sixty and older, women who had the lowest blood levels of folate were *twice* as likely to be depressed compared to women with higher levels. The authors point out that this link persists in spite of fortification of food with folic acid.[15]

For depression, LMF is the folate of choice. Studies that use folic acid to treat depression generally have poor results. Not so with LMF.

In a study published in the *Journal of Clinical Psychiatry*, depressed people who didn't respond to SSRIs were given 15 mg per day of LMF for sixty days, followed by a placebo for thirty days. They significantly improved when they were taking LMF.[16]

In another study, 554 depressed patients received LMF either alone or in combination with their current medication. LMF reduced symptoms of depression by 59 percent—with almost half the patients achieving remission (in other words, no more depression).[17]

Of note, there were virtually no side effects from LMF in either of these studies.

Antidepressants work better with LMF. In a study from the University of North Carolina, Chapel Hill, and several other institutions, scientists analyzed the results of two studies that added LMF to an antidepressant regimen in people not responding to the drug. With the vitamin added, depressive symptoms eased.

"These studies support the use of L-methylfolate in an adjunctive [additional] treatment in patients with major depressive disorder not responding to antidepressant monotherapy," concluded the researchers in *Primary Care Companion in CNS Disorders*. The researchers also note LMF is particularly effective in people who are obese and have high levels of inflammatory biomarkers.[18]

And in a study published in *Pharmacopsychiatry*, a team of U.S. and Canadian researchers analyzed the results from nine studies on LMF and depression, involving more than 6,700 depressed patients. They found that adding LMF to an antidepressant was 25 percent more effective than taking an antidepressant alone.[19]

Why is LMF more effective than folic acid?

It often comes down to your genes. There is a genetic mutation that is incredibly common: a mutation of the MTHFR gene, which provides instructions to the enzyme *methylenetetrahydrofolate reductase*, which in turn is responsible for the conversion of folic acid into LMF. In other words, if you have this genetic mutation, your body can't produce LMF, the form of folate that helps create serotonin, dopamine, and norepinephrine. And you're much more likely to be depressed.

That's why I order the MTHFR genetic test for *every* depressed patient I see. It's a simple test, involving an easy, painless cheek swab. If the test is positive, the patient needs to take at least 3 mg per day of LMF. I recommend L-5-MTHF, or Metafolin, the most effective, brain-friendly type of LMF. In fact, folic acid—the synthetic form of folate found in most supplements—actually *blocks* L-5-MTHF from entering the brain.

As for other folate tests: they're not particularly reliable. Standard tests for serum and RBC levels of folate are consistently inaccurate. Alternatively, checking MTHFR genetic variants *and* homocysteine levels (high homocysteine may be caused by low folate) are the best ways to determine folate status.

Getting enough folate. Folate-rich foods include asparagus, citrus fruits, fortified cereals, leafy green vegetables like spinach, and legumes (peas, beans, and lentils). But if you have a folate deficiency—especially if you have MTHFR variants, or high homocysteine—you probably need to supplement your diet with folate.

Historically, folic acid has been the main form in supplements. But as we've been discussing, it requires enzymatic transformation to the more active form of folate—a transformation that can be blocked by MTHFR gene variants. To prevent this problem, and to maximize therapeutic benefits, I recommend supplementation with LMF, starting at 2 mg daily. If after two weeks, there's no improvement, increase by 1 mg. Continue to increase every two weeks until you reach 5 mg. The protocol:

Step #1: Start with 2 mg, for two weeks.

Step #2: If no improvement after two weeks, increase to 4 mg.

Understanding the MTHFR Genetic Test

What is a genetic variant or mutation?

People typically have two copies of every gene—two "recipes" containing instructions for the creation of a functional compound like a protein. In the cellular process of being copied and rewritten, these "recipes" can sometimes accumulate errors—called mutations, variants, or *single nucleotide polymorphisms* (SNPs). Genes with one mutation are called *heterozygous*. Genes with two mutations are called *homozygous*. When there are mutations, one or both "recipes" of a given gene are fundamentally altered. And just as a dish made from a recipe that contains errors won't taste quite right, proteins manufactured from a mutated genetic code may be partially or completely dysfunctional.

There are several common MTHFR mutations that genetic testing can identify.

The two normal MTHFR genes are C677C and A1298A. For C677C, normal enzyme activity is labeled *CC*; a heterozygous mutation that leads to slightly reduced activity is labeled *CT*; and a homozygous mutation producing significantly reduced activity is labeled *TT*. For A1298A, normal activity is labeled *AA*; and a heterozygous mutation that produces generally reduced activity is labeled *CC*.

In the case of the MTHFR enzyme, the more mutations there are, the bigger the drop in the activity of the enzyme. A person who is TT, for example, has lost approximately 70 percent of their MTHFR activity.

Studies are starting to show that people with the MTHFR variant are more likely to be depressed. For example, a study in the journal *Cellular and Molecular Biology* showed that people with the TT variant were 37 percent more likely to be depressed than people without it.

Bottom line: MTHFR genetic testing is invaluable for determining folate requirements—and creating a supplementation plan.

Step #3: If no improvement after another two weeks, increase to 5 mg.

Step #4: If you don't see an improvement after four weeks of treatment, you may need more folate—up to 15 mg.

Alternatively—and more simply—you can take PureMelt B12 Folate, from Pure Encapsulations, using two pills daily.

There are a few cautions and precautions when supplementing with folate. Several medications and lifestyle choices can reduce folate levels: birth control pills, antiseizure medications, antacids, certain antibiotics, alcohol, and tobacco.

And if you take folate, you *must* take vitamin B12, because taking

Antidepressants Didn't Work— But Folate Did

I have seen thousands of depressed patients who didn't improve with antidepressant medications. Laboratory tests inevitably reveal multiple nutritional deficiencies—and the genetic mutation of the MTHFR gene, which blocks the formation of LMF, the form of folate that creates the neurotransmitters serotonin, dopamine, and norepinephrine.

Charlie was one of those patients—a twenty-two-year-old graduate student who had struggled with depression during his college years, but who was now suffering from an episode so severe he left school and returned home. Charlie had taken many different kinds of antidepressants, and also ketamine. But nothing provided consistent, long-lasting relief.

Testing showed that Charlie had a TT mutation of the MTHFR gene. He was put on a daily 3 mg dose of LMF.

Within three months, Charlie was able to return to school. He continued to take Celexa (citalopram), with the folate boosting its antidepressant effect, leading to dramatic improvement.

folate by itself can mask a vitamin B12 deficiency—a deficiency that can cause long-term nerve damage.

In my clinical experience, supplementing with folate occasionally causes agitation and anxiety. That's why I use the "start low and go slow" model—beginning with a dose of 2 mg per day and gradually increasing.

Thiamine (Vitamin B1)

In the brain, thiamine is involved with the release of the neurotransmitter acetylcholine, which plays a role in learning and memory, sleep, pain levels, the processing of sensory information, and muscle movement and control.

Thiamine deficiency is linked to neurodegenerative diseases like Alzheimer's and Parkinson's, and thiamine supplements can help both conditions.

And in my clinical experience, deficiency isn't uncommon. It can be caused by celiac disease, inflammatory bowel disease, bariatric surgery, anorexia, alcoholism, and a poor diet loaded with ultra-processed foods (UPFs) like refined carbohydrates.

Several studies link thiamine and depression.

How to induce depression? Stop the intake of thiamine. In a classic study from 1957 in the *American Journal of Clinical Nutrition*, scientists removed thiamine from the diet of men for fifteen to twenty-seven days—and all of the men developed depression (along with vomiting, muscle weakness, and loss of appetite). When thiamine was restored, the men recovered completely—starting with better mood and better appetite.[20]

Low thiamine, low mood. Chinese scientists studied more than 1,500 people aged fifty to seventy, looking at thiamine levels and depression. People with the lowest levels of thiamine were three times more likely to be depressed than people with the highest levels. There's a clear link between "poorer thiamine nutritional status and higher odds of depressive symptoms," wrote the researchers in the *Journal of Nutrition*.[21]

Thiamine vs. Alzheimer's

Thiamine is so protective of the brain that it may even help prevent Alzheimer's.

Neuroscientists have theorized that low levels of thiamine block the brain's ability to use glucose for fuel, leading to neurodegeneration—and Alzheimer's. In laboratory research, they found that benfotiamine—a synthetic form of fat-soluble thiamine that boosts blood levels 100 times greater than natural thiamine—could prevent the amyloid plaques and tau tangles linked to the brain disease.

In 2015, the first human research was conducted on benfotiamine, on seventy people with cognitive decline and Alzheimer's. The study showed significant slowing of mental decline compared to people getting a placebo.

Now, the thiamine-based drug is being studied in a nationwide clinical trial on four hundred people, aged fifty to eighty-nine, with cognitive decline and Alzheimer's. "Benfotiamine may do a much better job targeting the root cause of Alzheimer's compared to recently approved drugs for the disease," said Gary Gibson, PhD, a professor of neuroscience at the Feil Family Brain and Mind Research Institute at Weill Cornell Medicine in New York, and a lead researcher on the study. I'm pretty sure the results will bear him out.[22]

More thiamine, better mood. In a study published in the journal *Neuropsychobiology*, researchers from England found that low blood levels of thiamine were linked to "poor mood" in women—and taking a multivitamin with thiamine boosted blood levels and improved mood.[23]

Well-being restored. Researchers at the University of California, Davis, studied eighty older women with low levels of thiamine, giving half of them 10 mg of thiamine daily and half a placebo. Those receiving the thiamine supplement had a significant increase in "general well-being," wrote the researchers in the *Journal of Gerontology*. The women also had better appetite, ate more, gained weight, felt less fatigued, and slept better. The researchers recommend testing for thiamine levels in older people with depression (and with poor appetite, weight loss, fatigue, and sleep disorders).[24]

Thiamine for a clearer mind. Researchers gave 120 women either 50 mg of thiamine per day or a placebo. Those taking the thiamine were "more clearheaded, composed and energetic," and reaction times were faster.[25]

In a section on thiamine that I wrote for my textbook *Integrative Therapies for Depression*, I concluded that there is scientific evidence showing supplementing the diet with thiamine can improve mood, and that improvements in depressive symptoms are linked to increased blood levels of thiamine in people who had low levels *and* normal levels.

Good food sources of thiamine include beef, pork, shellfish, seeds, legumes, whole grains, and vegetables like spinach, brussels sprouts, asparagus, peas, and acorn squash.

For thiamine supplementation—in fact, for getting a therapeutic, brain-healing dose of *all* the B vitamins—I recommend B-Complex Plus, from Pure Encapsulations. It supplies all the B vitamins, including 100 mg of thiamine. If you've got a vitamin B12 or folate deficiency, you should add PureMelt B12 Folate, a product I discussed earlier in this chapter. If you follow the folate protocol I described above, use 1 mg pills of LMF.

Niacin (Vitamin B3)

In the early part of the twentieth century, half of all patients in psychiatric hospitals in the American South had *pellagra*, a disease that included schizophrenic-like psychosis among its many symptoms. The pioneering Joseph Goldberg, MD, theorized that a nutritional deficiency was behind the disease—and gave pellagra patients a varied diet of nutrient-dense, fresh food. Pellagra rates plummeted—and many formerly psychotic patients walked out the doors of institutions under their own authority and power, having been cured by diet.

About fifteen years later, the vitamin *niacin* was isolated—and niacin deficiency was identified as the culprit in pellagra.

In the decades that followed, pioneers in "orthomolecular psychiatry"—the use of nutrition to treat mental disorders—focused on niacin deficiency as the key cause of schizophrenia, laying the groundwork for the study of abnormal brain chemistry in mental health. Those pioneers included Abram Hoffer, MD, PhD, and the psychiatrist William Kaufman, MD. In the 1940s, Kaufman described "niacinamide nutritional deficiency disease" (niacinamide is another form of vitamin B3), enumerating symptoms like restlessness, irritability, mental sluggishness, excessive worry, insomnia, and persistent anxiety. In other words, Dr. Kaufman said his patients had symptoms linked to niacin even when they didn't have the outright niacin deficiency of pellagra—a groundbreaking insight at the time.

That "origin story" of niacin gives you a feel for the role of this vitamin in mental health: If you're getting too little niacin, you're at risk for poor mental health. In fact, for poor health, period.

More than four hundred enzymes—the spark plugs of biochemical activity—depend on niacin. The vitamin is a must for producing adenosine triphosphate (ATP), the basic fuel for every cell in the body. Niacin allows genes to activate and "express" themselves. It repairs DNA. It ensures cell-to-cell signaling. It helps synthesize cholesterol and fatty acids. And niacin supports antioxidants in cleaning up the "free radicals" that damage cellular health.

But back to mental health for a moment. Niacin:

- regulates levels of the neurotransmitter dopamine;

- helps with the synthesis of other neurotransmitters, like histamine and acetylcholine;

- is a precursor for nicotinamide adenine dinucleotide (NAD), which supports many functions in the brain, including the survival of neurons, the ability of neurons to change and adapt (plasticity), and the reduction of oxidative stress;

- increases blood flow to and in the brain; and

- increases BDNF, which is a must for brain health.

As Dr. Hoffer put it, "If all the vitamin B3 were removed from our food, everyone would become psychotic within one year." Scientific research shows niacin might also help prevent and treat depression and bipolar disorder.

Less likely to be depressed. In a study of nearly eighteen thousand people, those with the highest intake of dietary niacin were 35 percent less likely to be depressed than those with the lowest intake. The study was published in the April 2023 issue of the *International Journal of Vitamin and Nutrition Research.*[26]

No poststroke depression. A study in the January 2018 issue of *Clinical Nutrition Research* showed that stroke patients with high dietary intakes of niacin were far less likely to become depressed and anxious.[27]

Bipolar disorder—improved with niacin. In a scientific paper in the January 27, 2018, issue of *Nutrients*, a doctor at the prestigious Karolinska Institute in Stockholm reports the case history of a patient with bipolar type 2 disorder who was taking lithium and other medications but without much benefit. But when the patient started taking nicotinic acid (a form of niacin), he "experienced a comparatively strong effect"— and "slowly it was discovered that the patient could lower and cease all medications except for nicotinic acid." The patient remained "stable and calm" during eleven years of the vitamin, at a dose of 1 gram, three times per day. If he stopped taking nicotinic acid, however, he became depressed and anxious within two to three days—but he was restored to good mental health within a day of resuming the vitamin.[28]

There are two possible regimens for getting enough niacin. Take B-Complex Plus, from Pure Encapsulations—which includes niacin—following the dosage recommendation on the label. Or take niacinamide, 500 mg, two times daily. In my clinical experience, additional niacinamide can be helpful in easing the irritability and anxiety that often accompany depression.

B Vitamins

Use this practical, step-by-step summary to implement the therapeutic actions discussed in this chapter.

Vitamin B12

Step #1: Take a B12 test.

Step #2: Consider testing for homocysteine. If the level is high (above 12), it's more likely you have a B12 deficiency.

Step #3: Consider testing for MMA, a breakdown product of amino acids. If the level is high (above 245 nmol/L), it's likely you need more B12 or have an outright deficiency. (Steps #2 and #3 are *supportive* testing, to give you and your health care professional the clearest idea about your B12 levels and need for supplementation.)

Step #4: If B12 levels are under 500 pg/mL, supplement with B12, by injection or sublingually (under the tongue). (Please see the discussion about B12 testing for more information about this recommendation.)

Step #5: Receive B12 injections. The best forms are: *hydroxocobalamin*, which is a precursor to the active form of B12; and *methylcobalamin*, which is the active form of B12 that is used by the tissues of the body.

I recommend injections two times per week for one month, testing one week after the last injection.

Step #6: If you prefer not to take injections, start with oral supplementation, using methylcobalamin. Take a daily dose of 2,000 mcg, twice per day. Take it in "sublingual" form—a dissolvable pill placed under the tongue, where B12 can be absorbed easily and quickly. The sublingual B12 I recommend is PureMelt B12 Folate, from Pure Encapsulations.

Step #7: Consider eating more B12-rich food, like beef, fish, chicken, eggs, milk, cheese, and yogurt.

Folate (vitamin B9)

Step #1: Take an MTHFR genetic test, a simple test usually involving an easy, painless cheek swab.

Step #2: Consider testing for homocysteine, an amino acid that can act as a neurotoxin. High levels of homocysteine are consistently linked to low levels of folate.

Step #3: If the MTHFR test is positive for any variant—indicating a genetic mutation that blocks the creation of LMF, the active form of the vitamin—you need to start taking at least 2 mg per day of LMF. Gradually increase the dosage until you feel symptoms are stabilized.

I recommend L-5-MTHF, or Metafolin, the most effective, brain-friendly type of LMF. (Folic acid—the synthetic form of folate found in most supplements—actually blocks L-5-MTHF from entering the brain.)

Another, simpler alternative regimen: Take PureMelt B12 Folate, from Pure Encapsulations, taking two pills daily.

Step #4: Eat more folate-rich foods. They include asparagus, citrus fruits, fortified cereals, leafy green vegetables like spinach, and legumes (peas, beans, and lentils).

Thiamine (vitamin B1)

Step #1: Consider taking a thiamine supplement if you have any one of the following risk factors: celiac disease; inflammatory bowel disease; bariatric surgery; anorexia; alcoholism; or a poor diet loaded with UPFs like refined carbohydrates.

For thiamine, I recommend taking B-Complex Plus, from Pure Encapsulations, which delivers brain-healthy doses of all the B vitamins, with 100 mg of thiamine per capsule. Take one capsule per day, with a meal.

Step #2: Eat more thiamine-rich foods, including beef, pork, shellfish, seeds, legumes, whole grains, and vegetables like spinach, brussels sprouts, asparagus, peas, and acorn squash.

Niacin (vitamin B3)

Step #1: For adequate niacin, take B-Complex Plus, from Pure Encapsulations.

Step #2: If depressed *and* anxious, add niacinamide, 500 mg, twice daily, with meals.

CHAPTER 7

Minerals

Key Elements of Mental Well-Being

> Zinc, magnesium, chromium, iron, and
> other minerals are musts for mental health.

s your health rock solid? And when I say "rock," I mean it *literally*.

There are sixteen essential minerals in your diet, from calcium and chromium to magnesium and zinc. These bioactive minerals are ultimately derived from rock. And without sufficient minerals, your health won't have a solid foundation. For example:

Magnesium is a must for strong bones and teeth. *Zinc* boosts the power of your immune system. *Chromium* balances blood sugar. *Iron* maintains the integrity of oxygen-carrying red blood cells (RBCs).

Essential minerals are also important cofactors that help enzymes spark thousands of different reactions in the body, from the creation of the cellular fuel adenosine triphosphate (ATP) to the clotting of blood.

Minerals are also important in the brain, where they help regulate neurotransmitters, which control signaling from neuron to neuron. Minerals control how neurotransmitters like serotonin, dopamine, and norepinephrine are made, how they are released, and how they travel across the tiny gaps between neurons called synapses. Minerals also maintain the integrity of the synapses themselves. And they control the production of hormones that influence brain function.

But many minerals have gone AWOL from the American diet.

Tens of millions of Americans probably have what health experts call a "subclinical deficiency" of one or more essential minerals: not an outright deficiency that causes obvious deficiency-related symptoms, but a very low level that slowly undermines health and eventually shows up as a chronic health problem. Like depression.

Minerals are missing for several reasons. Our soil has been depleted for decades by intensive commercial farming. (One study found that mineral levels in food plunged 84 percent from 1940 to 2002.[1]) Pesticides can block the uptake of minerals by plants. Minerals are stripped out of highly processed foods. The sugar in many highly processed foods forces minerals out of the body. Many over-the-counter and prescription pharmaceuticals block the uptake of minerals by the brain. And stress and chronic disease drain the body of minerals.

> **Bottom line:** Minerals have gone missing—and
> rising levels of depression may be the result.

Along with affecting neurotransmitters, there are many other factors linking minerals and depression:

Low brain-derived neurotrophic factor (BDNF). The minerals zinc, magnesium, and lithium influence the genetic expression and activity of BDNF, which helps neurons grow and adapt. People with depression often have low levels of BDNF.

Hyperactive N-methyl-D-aspartate (NMDA). Zinc and magnesium help calm neuroreceptors for NMDA. When these receptors are overstimulated, so are neurons—leading to the neuroinflammation that is linked to depression.

Less inflammation. Neuroinflammation and depression go hand in hand. Antioxidant minerals like zinc, copper, magnesium, and iron help cool neuroinflammation. But if minerals are missing, they can be replaced with targeted nutritional supplementation—reversing depression.

Let's look at the minerals that are most important to treating depression, starting with zinc.

(One mineral we won't be looking at in this chapter is lithium. It's such an important depression fighter that I've devoted an entire chapter to it, Chapter 8.)

Think Zinc

Zinc is a so-called "trace mineral"—your body needs it in very small amounts of less than 20 milligrams (mg) a day. But those small amounts make a big difference in your body and brain—particularly when it comes to depression. The scientific evidence linking zinc and depression is very strong.

Zinc-rich diets lower the risk of depression. In a study of more than two thousand middle-aged and older adults, Australian researchers found that those with the highest dietary intake of zinc were 30 to 50 percent less likely to develop depression compared to those with the lowest intake. (The best food sources of zinc are oysters, red meat, eggs, wheat germ, spinach, pumpkin and squash seeds, nuts, chocolate, chicken, beans, and mushrooms.)[2]

Thirty-three percent lower zinc in depressed people. In a study in the *Journal of Affective Disorders,* Polish researchers found that zinc levels in depressed people were on average 22 percent lower than in healthy people.[3] In a similar study, published in *Biological Trace Element Research*, depressed people had blood levels of zinc 25 percent lower than healthy people.[4]

Zinc beats depression. Japanese researchers studied thirty women, dividing them into two groups: one group was given a multivitamin, and one group was given a multivitamin *and* zinc. After ten weeks, the women taking zinc had a big increase in zinc levels—and a big decrease in depression and anger. The women taking only the multivitamin had no increase in zinc—and no decrease in depression. "Zinc supplementation may be effective in reducing anger and depression," wrote the researchers in the *European Journal of Clinical Nutrition.*[5]

Overweight and depressed—until they took zinc. People with depression are almost twice as likely to be obese as people who aren't depressed. In a study published in the March 2020 issue of *Nutrition*, researchers gave 125 depressed people who were also obese or overweight various combinations of supplements and placebos—and found zinc was the most effective treatment for easing depressive symptoms.[6]

Multiple sclerosis (MS) patients with depression benefit from zinc. Depression is common in people with MS. In a study published in *Pharmacological Reports*, depressed MS patients who took zinc had less depression after twelve weeks, compared to little or no change in those taking a placebo.[7]

Zinc boosts the power of antidepressant meds. Researchers in Australia analyzed the results from four studies in which a zinc supplement was added to an antidepressant. "Zinc significantly lowered depressive symptom scores of depressive patients," wrote the researchers, in the *Journal of Affective Disorders.*[8]

In fact, one mechanism of action of antidepressants is that they increase blood levels of zinc.

Zinc, a biomarker for depression. In a study intended to be a definitive statement about the effect of zinc on depression, Polish researchers in psychiatry, pharmacology, chemistry, and medicine studied 164 people (sixty-nine currently depressed; forty-five in remission; and fifty healthy).[9] They concluded:

- zinc levels are much lower in depressed people than in healthy people;

- the lower the level of zinc, the more depressive episodes in a twelve-month period;

- when depressed people are in remission, their zinc levels are the same as healthy people; and

- depressed people who are resistant to antidepressant medication have lower levels of zinc.

"Serum zinc concentration might be considered as a potential biomarker of major depressive disorder," concluded the researchers, in *Metabolic Brain Disease*. Put another way: Optimizing zinc levels is an important step in treating depression.

Zinc probably works in many ways, including: calming NMDA receptors in the brain; and increasing levels of BDNF. (Zinc affects BDNF in several ways: activating its genetic expression, helping form the BDNF molecule, and improving BDNF signaling.)

Likewise, the neurotransmitter dopamine depends on zinc—not only for making dopamine, but also for slowing dopamine "reuptake" in the neuron, which allows dopamine levels to rise.

Testing to find out if you're low in zinc is a challenge, both in getting accurate results and interpreting them. But if you're depressed you probably don't need zinc testing—because it's very likely you need more zinc. (It's also likely you have a deficiency if you have frequent infections, white spots on your nails, a weakened sense of taste and lack of enjoyment in food, or you're a senior. Zinc deficiency is also common in adolescents, when puberty creates an increased demand.)

If you're a depressed adult, I recommend 60 mg of zinc per day, 30 mg two times daily, with meals. (Zinc supplements can cause gastrointestinal upset if taken on an empty stomach.) Once you're in remission, take 30 mg per day, 15 mg two times daily, with meals.

But if you take more than 40 mg of zinc per day for an extended period of time, you need to monitor copper levels, as high levels of zinc can eventually cause copper levels to go too low. Let's explore this zinc-copper connection in depth.

Copper:
Too Much of a Good Thing?

The essential minerals zinc and copper are like a nutritional seesaw: if the level of one goes up, the level of the other goes down. High zinc, low copper. High copper, low zinc. And while a tiny amount of copper is a must for good health, more copper is not necessarily a good thing.

In the body, the copper molecule is found in the form of positively charged *copper ions* that can easily turn into *free radicals*—unstable molecules that oxidize and damage cells—including brain cells.

Extra copper has been linked to many mental disorders, including schizophrenia, general anxiety disorder, obsessive-compulsive disorder, bipolar disorder—and depression.

And Wilson's disease, a genetic disease that leads to an accumulation of copper in the body, has many psychiatric symptoms, including temper tantrums, inability to focus and concentrate, loss of emotional control, insomnia—and depression.

Excess copper also creates an excess of dopamine and its partner norepinephrine, causing symptoms like irritability and agitation. And high copper blocks the neurotransmission of gamma-aminobutyric acid (GABA), a neurotransmitter that helps regulate anxiety, stress, sleep, and pain.

Bottom line: Extra copper *imbalances* the biochemistry of the brain, causing or contributing to depression.

Many studies link excess copper and depression.

When copper is up, you feel down. Many studies show that copper levels in people with depression are much higher than in people who don't have depression, according to research published in *Frontiers in Neuroscience* in 2023. In one study, people with higher copper levels had an 85 percent higher risk of depression compared to people with normal levels. In another, half of all patients with depression had higher levels of copper.[10]

Researchers from China reviewed the results from twenty-one other studies on copper and depression, involving more than 2,400 depressed and nondepressed people, publishing their results in *Psychiatry Research*. "Patients with depression had higher blood levels of copper" than people without depression, they concluded—a link so strong, they said, that copper could be a "biomarker" for depression.[11] Just like zinc—with other scientists saying too *little* zinc is a biomarker for depression; and these scientists saying too *much* copper is also a biomarker.

There are two ways to know for certain that you have excess copper and low zinc: testing for plasma zinc and copper; and the Trace Mineral Hair Analysis, a hair test that measures zinc and copper levels.

With results in hand, your doctor can definitively determine whether or not you have excess copper and low zinc. And if you do, there's a

The Strange Case of
Too Little Copper

The trace mineral copper is a perfect illustration of the "Goldilocks Principle"—you can get too little, you can get too much, but you need the "just right" amount.

The "just right" amount of copper is an ally of good health, helping to regulate immunity, balance blood sugar, make hormones, and produce red blood cells. It's also key in the creation of neurotransmitters.

But both *too much* and *too little* copper can cause depression. Too much typically causes an agitated depression, with irritability and mood swings. Too little causes depression with lack of motivation and fatigue.

I commonly see copper deficiency and depression in people overdoing it on zinc supplements, and in people who have celiac disease and inflammatory bowel disease, both of which reduce the absorption of nutrients.

In a case history of low copper levels, published in the journal *Cureus,* a man with quadriplegia was taking high levels of zinc as part of his wound care regimen—and ended up in the ER with breathing difficulties, and severe constipation. Testing showed he had severe anemia, a low white blood cell count (leukopenia)—and his copper levels were below 10 micrograms per deciliter (mcg/dL). Normal levels are 70 to 140.[12]

His zinc supplementation was stopped, and he started on copper supplementation. After three months, the anemia and leukopenia had cleared up.

Bottom line: Zinc supplementation is almost always a plus if you have depression—but don't take too much! If you have celiac disease or inflammatory bowel disease, ask your doctor to check your zinc-copper balance.

straightforward, simple way to treat the problem: take zinc, at the doses recommended in this chapter. But remember:

Zinc is a mineral, not a fast-acting medication. It can take three to four months for zinc supplementation to restore a normal zinc-copper balance.

Magnanimous Magnesium

Magnesium is arguably *the* most generous mineral in your body, bestowing its benefits on every cell, tissue, organ, and system.

Magnesium plays a role in more than three hundred enzyme systems, the biochemical spark plugs that ignite and direct cellular activity. As a cofactor, magnesium is way more active than any other nutrient, mineral, or vitamin.

For example, if magnesium is in short supply, so is ATP, the fundamental fuel that powers every cell. Too little magnesium also means your blood sugar isn't regulated, your immune system is weakened, your ability to handle stress is blunted, and—most importantly for people with depression—your *sleep* is compromised.

How does too little magnesium cause mayhem in the brain? Several ways:

Neurotransmitters. Magnesium plays a key role in the formation of neurotransmitters. If magnesium levels are suboptimal, you're likely to have imbalanced levels of two neurotransmitters: mood-regulating *serotonin* and pleasure-supplying *dopamine*. Plus, magnesium does more than help maintain serotonin levels—it also helps the neurotransmitter bind to neurons and transmit signals.

BDNF. Magnesium is important for maintaining and raising levels of BDNF, a compound that is critical for the development of new, healthy neurons, and for *plasticity*, the ability of neurons to adapt to new inputs and situations.

NDMA receptors. Low levels of magnesium release the brakes on NDMA receptors, and the unchecked receptors can overexcite neurons, causing damage (and even death).

Stress hormones. The mineral helps regulate the release of neuron-damaging stress hormones in the brain.

Unfortunately, most of us get too little magnesium in our diets—with research showing that three out of four Americans get less than the recommended dietary allowance (RDA). That statistic matches my experience with patients, where magnesium deficiency is *the most common deficiency* that I encounter.

Magnesium deficiency is so common because modern life is very tough on magnesium.

Ultra-processed foods (UPFs)—like sugary drinks, fast food, packaged snacks, and processed meats—comprise about 60 percent of calories in the typical American diet; and UPFs are *very* low in magnesium.

Mechanized, commercial farming has stripped the soil of magnesium—so even if you're eating a diet rich in whole foods like fruits, vegetables, and whole grains, you still might not be getting the magnesium you need.

Alcohol and caffeine block the absorption of magnesium and increase urinary excretion.

Medications can rob the body of magnesium, like proton pump inhibitors (PPIs) for heartburn, diuretics, and some antibiotics. Fifteen million Americans take a prescription PPI like Nexium, Prilosec, and Prevacid—and another thirty-five million regularly take over-the-counter PPIs.

Chronic health conditions like type 2 diabetes and kidney disease can decrease magnesium absorption. So can celiac disease, which commonly causes deficiencies in *all* the minerals discussed in this chapter. Gastric bypass can also reduce the absorption of magnesium and other minerals.

Chronic stress is an almost universal problem in our 24/7 society, where our to-do list is always trying to catch up with the clock—and chronic stress drains the body of magnesium. In one study, researchers found that chronic stress produced "significant decreases" in both blood magnesium and total magnesium. "These findings support the need for magnesium supplementation for people living in conditions of chronic stress," they concluded.

And there's plenty of scientific evidence showing that low levels of magnesium can make you feel down—and that adding magnesium can reverse depression.

Scientific support

Interestingly, the first scientific report of treating depression with magnesium was way back in 1921, with success in 220 of 250 cases, according to a scientific paper in *Medical Hypothesis*—making magnesium the first antidepressant. The report goes on to say that "there is more than sufficient evidence to implicate inadequate dietary magnesium as the main cause of treatment-resistant depression (TRD)—and that physicians should prescribe magnesium for TRD . . . and for nearly all depressives."

I couldn't agree more. Now let's look at some recent scientific studies.

More magnesium, less depression. In a review of eleven studies on magnesium and depression, Chinese scientists found that a higher dietary intake of magnesium reduced the risk of depression by 43 percent—and that low magnesium blood levels increased the risk of depression by 19 percent.[13]

In similar research, Italian scientists looked at eighteen scientific studies on magnesium and depression, and found a strong link between low blood levels of magnesium and depression. They also found that supplementing the diet with magnesium improved depressive symptoms. "Supplementation with magnesium" could be beneficial for depression, they concluded, in the June 3, 2020, issue of *Nutrients*.[14]

And in a meta-analysis, published in 2023, researchers analyzed the results of seven studies on magnesium and depression, involving 323 people, finding the mineral caused a "significant decline in depression."[15]

Beating depression in type 2 diabetes—with magnesium. Diabetes *doubles* the risk of depression, with up to 33 percent of people with type 2 diabetes affected by depression, according to a study in the *Journal of Affective Disorders*.[16] Adding magnesium might help—a lot.

Mexican researchers gave either magnesium or an antidepressant to twenty-three older women with type 2 diabetes who had low magnesium levels, and who were depressed. They found that magnesium was just as effective as the drug in relieving depressive symptoms.[17]

Do you have low magnesium?

Are low levels of magnesium affecting your brain? Finding out isn't easy.

Blood magnesium levels do *not* reveal deficiencies—because 99 percent of magnesium is found in the bones, muscles, heart, and liver, with only 1 percent in the blood.

In my clinical experience, trace mineral hair analysis provides a simple, affordable, and useful tool for identifying magnesium deficiency.

There are also several clinical indicators of magnesium deficiency, including anxiety, insomnia, constipation, and health conditions that involve muscle spasms (asthma, muscle cramps, migraines, eye twitching, etc.).

But even without testing, I recommend a magnesium supplement for *every* patient with depression—because deficiency is so prevalent; and because magnesium is so safe and effective.

But don't forget about increasing magnesium in your diet, too. The best sources are spinach and other dark-green leafy vegetables, potatoes, beans, nuts and seeds, yogurt, oatmeal, brown rice, avocados, halibut, and wheat bran.

The many types of magnesium

There are many different forms of supplemental magnesium, like magnesium glycinate, magnesium oxide, magnesium citrate, and magnesium gluconate. In my clinical experience, all of them are equally effective, with one exception: magnesium oxide, which is poorly absorbed.

Some health experts recommend magnesium L-threonate as the best form of magnesium for the brain. That's because a few studies show brain-based benefits, like healthier brain cells and protection against age-related mental decline. There's nothing wrong with magnesium L-threonate, but it is more expensive than the other forms.

One more point: some people *may* respond better to one form of magnesium versus another, so it can be worthwhile to switch forms to maximize benefits.

Finally Hopeful Success Story

PATIENT: Donald
TREATMENT FOR: Severe depression

Donald was a forty-two-year-old with severe, long-standing depression that hadn't responded to treatment with antidepressants, including Prozac (fluoxetine), Cymbalta (duloxetine), or Lexapro (escitalopram). His marriage was unhappy. He felt overwhelmed at work. And he had gained weight, a common side effect of antidepressants.

When I saw Donald, he was taking a daily dose of extended release Seroquel XR (quetiapine, 150 mg), Zoloft (sertraline, 100 mg), and Wellbutrin (bupropion, 150 mg). He told me that the medications had initially seemed to "take the edge off"—but they weren't working any longer.

His goals for treatment were to reduce his medications—not only because their effectiveness had declined over time, but because he had gained weight.

The first thing I did was give him a round of tests, to detect important deficiencies and imbalances.

He had several problems, including: Imbalances in his gut microbiome, revealed by the Organic Acid Test. The MTHFR genetic variant CT, which interferes with the absorption of folic acid and other B vitamins. Kryptopyrrole, which depletes the body of zinc and vitamin C. Low levels of magnesium.

I supplemented with daily doses of: Probiotics (for the gut microbiome). The B vitamins methylfolate (3 mg) and vitamin B6 (50 mg). Zinc (60 mg). And magnesium glycinate (480 mg).

After three months, Donald's depressive symptoms had slowly but steadily improved. At that point, we began to slowly reduce or eliminate some of his medications.

At six months, Donald said he was very happy with his progress—with the emphasis on *happy*. He was no longer taking Seroquel, and the doses of the other drugs had been reduced. Work had become more manageable. He had lost weight. And his wife said that she had rediscovered the man she had fallen in love with.

Best type, best dose

I typically recommend a dose of 240 mg, twice per day, either in the form of magnesium glycinate or magnesium citrate.

If you take magnesium threonate, the dose is 1,000 mg (which delivers 72 mg of elemental magnesium), twice per day.

The main side effect from taking magnesium is loose stools. This laxative effect is most common with magnesium oxide, another reason not to use it. If you develop loose stools, split or decrease the dose, or switch to a time-released, long-acting form of magnesium.

Chromium:
Custom Treatment for Atypical Depression

That special, rust-resistant shine on stainless steel knives, forks, and spoons is produced by a coating of chromium. But don't worry. There are *many* forms of chromium, including the kind used in stainless steel (hexavalent chromium), and the kind your body uses to stay healthy (trivalent chromium).

In the four decades since scientists discovered that trivalent chromium is an essential nutrient, they've discovered quite a few other facts about the mineral, including:

You're probably not getting enough chromium in your diet. Researchers estimate that nine out of ten Americans are low in chromium—particularly seniors, and people who eat a lot of sugary food.

Chromium is a must for metabolic balance. Chromium stabilizes glucose (blood sugar) and insulin (the hormone that ushers blood sugar out of the bloodstream and into the cells)—thereby helping prevent type 2 diabetes. Our low intake of chromium is probably one of the reasons why thirty-four million Americans are diabetic, and another eighty-eight million are prediabetic.

Chromium is stabilizing in more ways than one. It also stabilizes cholesterol and triglyceride, heart-hurting blood fats. It stabilizes body weight, by helping you build calorie-burning muscle and shed fat. And it can stabilize *mood*—in fact, its ability to stabilize insulin *and* mood might rely on the same mechanism of action: the regulation of Glucose Transporter 4 (GLUT4).

GLUT4 is a protein that helps glucose find its way out of the bloodstream and into muscle and fat cells. Chromium *activates* GLUT4, and it *positions* GLUT4 on the cellular membrane (outer covering), where it can do its job.

What does that have to do with mood? Well, your mood-controlling brain is a glucose fiend: the brain is 2 percent of the body's weight, but consumes 20 percent of the body's supply of glucose. And not surprisingly, scientists have discovered that chromium-dependent GLUT4 plays a role in the brain.

In the hippocampus—a part of the brain critical to memory—a reduction in GLUT4 stunts the connections between neurons, slowing activity. That leads to the emotional symptoms of depression, like sadness, apathy, and guilt. And to cognitive problems, like poor concentration and memory. Experts say GLUT4 dysfunction may explain the glaring link between diabetes and depression—with up to 50 percent of people with diabetes suffering from this mood disorder. (The condition is so common it has its own name: *diabetic distress.*)

Clinical studies confirm the chromium/depression connection—particularly in so-called "atypical depression," which often involves overeating and weight gain.

Beneficial effect on atypical depression and seasonal affective disorder (SAD). In a paper from the Depression Clinical and Research Program at Harvard Medical School, researchers point out that chromium has a "beneficial effect" on atypical depression, and SAD (depression during the darker days of fall and winter). They note the mineral is particularly effective at treating the overeating of atypical depression—probably because chromium balances both blood sugar and brain chemistry.[18]

And in a scientific paper from the departments of psychiatry, psychology, and medicine at the University of North Carolina, researchers theorize that chromium should be particularly effective in patients who have diabetes *and* depression *and* binge eating.[19]

Dramatic improvements in refractory depression. In a study from psychiatrists at the University of North Carolina School (where a lot of the chromium/depression research was conducted), doctors gave chromium supplements to eight patients with "refractory" (untreatable) depression. The patients had "dramatic improvements in their symptoms and functioning," wrote the psychiatrists in the *International Journal of Neuropsychopharmacology*. They theorized that chromium was so effective because it balanced insulin levels, made tryptophan (and therefore serotonin) more available, and improved the release of norepinephrine.[20]

Reduced mood symptoms in premenstrual dysphoric disorder (PMDD). Researchers gave chromium and/or an antidepressant to five women with PMDD—intense emotional symptoms like mood swings, depression, irritability, and anxiety during the week or two before menstruation. "Chromium treatment," they wrote in the *Journal of Dietary Supplements*, "reduced mood symptoms and improved overall health" in most of the women. In some cases, chromium worked on its own; in others, the combination of chromium and an antidepressant was more effective than either alone.[21]

Remission of symptoms in persistent depressive disorder (PDD). PDD takes a terrible toll on daily life, with long-lasting feelings of sadness and low mood. Doctors treated five people with refractory PDD with chromium, adding the mineral to their antidepressant medication. In every case, the patients had complete remission of their symptoms. When the doctors stopped the chromium and substituted other dietary supplements, the depression returned—confirming that it was the chromium causing the improvement.[22]

Promising antidepressant effects. In a study from researchers in the department of psychiatry and behavioral sciences at Duke University Medical Center in North Carolina, fifteen people with the atypical form of major depressive disorder were given either 600 micrograms (mcg) of chromium or a placebo for eight weeks. Seven out of ten people taking chromium had a positive response; people taking the placebo had no response.[23]

Beneficial for severe carbohydrate cravings. In a study of seventy-five people with atypical depression (most of whom were overweight or obese), those taking 600 mcg of chromium per day had "significant improvements" in symptoms—with a decrease in appetite, overeating, carbohydrate cravings, and mood swings during the day. "Chromium may be beneficial for patients with atypical depression who also have severe carbohydrate cravings," wrote the researchers in the *Journal of Psychiatric Practice.*[24]

Chromium is found in many everyday foods, like vegetables, meat, fish, bread, cereal, and beer. But the amount of chromium you get from the diet can't really touch a case of depression. For that, you need to supplement the diet with chromium—particularly since chromium is rapidly used up by high sugar intake, emotional stress, exercise, and infection.

If you are overweight or obese (70 percent of us are); have diabetes; have atypical depression, SAD, or PMDD—consider taking chromium.

Your physician might want to check your chromium level with a Trace Mineral Hair Analysis. If levels are low, you should definitely supplement your diet with chromium.

To supplement the diet with chromium and other trace minerals, I recommend a trace mineral supplement: Trace Minerals, from Pure Encapsulations. It contains 200 mcg of chromium, which is usually enough to restore normal levels and reduce or eliminate depressive symptoms.

Iron-Poor Brain?

Maybe you've heard of "iron-poor blood"—a phrase commonly used to describe a deficiency of the mineral that guarantees the integrity of *hemoglobin*, the molecule in red blood cells that carries oxygen throughout the body.

But have you heard of an iron-poor *brain?*

Yes, low iron intake is linked to poor mental development. And to emotional problems. Two examples of the connection:

1) Twice as many women as men are clinically depressed, a statistic that holds true from adolescence through childbearing age—the very years when menstruation, pregnancy, and lactation deplete a woman's body of iron.

2) Iron deficiency can cause anemia, a condition in which the body doesn't have enough healthy red blood cells. And anemia is strongly linked to depression (and apathy and fatigue, both symptoms of depression).

Iodine: First Aid for Your Thyroid

Iodine is a trace mineral that is found in ocean water and in soil, and is added to salt. Getting enough is a must.

The body uses iodine to create the thyroid hormones T3 and T4. The thyroid gland is your body's gas pedal, controlling how fast (or slow) everything moves. When thyroid hormones are low—a condition called hypothyroidism—everything slows way, way down.

Among many possible symptoms: you're tired during the day; you gain weight or can't seem to lose it; your muscles are stiff and achy; you feel cold all the time; memory and focus are poor; and you feel depressed.

In fact, 40 percent of people with hypothyroidism become clinically depressed, according to a scientific paper titled *Hypothyroidism and Depression*.

And, says the paper, an estimated 4 to 40 percent of people with subclinical hypothyroidism—low, but not officially deficient levels of thyroid hormones—are depressed.[25] More proof of the thyroid/depression connection: When thyroid hormone is added to antidepressant medication, responses are often better than with the medication alone, according to a study from the University of California, Los Angeles, published in the *Journal of Endocrinological Investigation*.[26]

For a small percentage of people with depression, simply bringing iodine up to an adequate level can go a long way to resolving depression. The supplement I recommend is Trace Minerals, from Pure Encapsulations, which delivers 100 mcg of iodine daily.

How does low iron cause depression? Scientists have a couple of ideas.

- Iron activates nitric oxide, a neurotransmitter. Nitric oxide also widens blood vessels in the brain, ensuring an adequate supply of oxygen.

- Iron balances the neurotransmitter glutamate, an "excitatory" neurotransmitter that can over-activate and overstimulate neurons.

- Iron is critical for the activity of GABA, an "inhibitory" neurotransmitter that calms neurons.

- Iron is a cofactor for tryptophan hydroxylase, which helps form serotonin, and for tyrosine hydroxylase, which helps form dopamine.

- Iron also plays an important role in *myelination*, the formation of protective insulation around nerve fibers, allowing for the efficient transmission of nerve impulses.

But whatever the cause or causes, scientific studies of people prove the emotional impact of low iron.

Double the risk of depression. A study in the *European Journal of Clinical Nutrition* involving 192 women found that those with low levels of ferritin—the stored form of iron—had *double* the risk of depression.[27]

Twenty-five percent less depressed—after taking iron. In a nine-month study from researchers at the University of Pennsylvania, anemic new mothers who received iron were 25 percent less likely to feel depressed, anxious, and stressed.[28]

Confirming the role of iron. And in a meta-analysis of three studies on iron and depression, published in *Psychiatry Research,* scientists found that people with low iron intake had a 43 percent increased risk of depression compared to people with high iron intake.[29]

Unfortunately, iron deficiency is *the* most common nutrient deficiency in the world. That's why it's good to eat iron-rich foods like meat, poultry, seafood, beans, and iron-fortified cereals.

But an iron-rich diet is *not* going to reverse iron-involved depression.

For that, you need an iron *supplement*. And it's best to take an iron supplement with a doctor's guidance, for several reasons.

One, iron should not be taken unless there is a test-proven deficiency. That's because it's possible to take too much iron, particularly in men and postmenopausal women, neither of whom has an ongoing means of disposing of excess iron, which can injure the heart and brain. So a doctor needs to carefully monitor dosing.

Two, lab work is a must to verify an iron deficiency. (However, it's important to note that depression linked to low iron can occur *before* blood levels are low enough for you to be officially considered "iron deficient.")

Three, there are many possible causes of iron deficiency aside from a low-iron diet, including colon cancer, celiac disease, and stomach ulcers. If you're iron deficient, you and your doctor need to determine the cause.

Bottom line: I recommend that everyone who is depressed (particularly women with heavy menstrual bleeding) be tested for iron and for ferritin. If levels of both iron and ferritin are low, you should eat more iron-rich foods *and* take iron-enhancing supplements.

I recommend supplementation with *ferrous bisglycinate*, a form of iron that doesn't cause the typical side effects of iron supplementation, which include constipation, nausea, and stomach upset. Take 28 mg, once per day, with meals. Add a supplement of 250 mg of vitamin C, to boost absorption.

The goal: iron levels higher than 50 grams per deciliter (g/dL), and ferritin levels close to 100 grams per liter (g/L). You should be retested three months after starting supplementation. Once iron levels have normalized, you can stop taking the supplement.

Iron Deficiency = Happiness Deficiency

The story of my thirty-five-year-old patient Kristen illustrates how iron deficiency can cause depression.

When I first saw Kristen in my office, she had severe depression, including persistent sadness, a lack of pleasure in any activity, feelings of worthlessness, problems getting to sleep and staying asleep, and anxiety. She told me that she had felt anxious since she was in her teens, but the depression had only started six months ago—when she moved to the United States from England, starting a job that turned out to be very stressful, and ending her long-term romantic relationship.

After her depressive symptoms began, Kristen saw a new primary care physician in the United States. She told him she was so depressed and anxious she couldn't get out of bed in the morning, and the doctor prescribed the antidepressant Zoloft, at 150 mg daily. At work, she requested and was granted a one-month medical leave. She also started weekly talk therapy, and the therapist recommended her to me.

At Kristen's first office visit, I conducted a history and physical, and diagnosed severe major depressive disorder (single episode), and generalized anxiety disorder. Kristen told me she had a history of anemia. I ordered baseline blood work, which had not been done for years.

Kristen's lab results indicated that she had iron deficiency without anemia. In other words, blood levels of iron were low, although her hemoglobin (the iron-carrying molecule in the blood) was still normal.

Kristen's Functional Psychiatry Treatment Plan included:

- Iron bisglycinate, 27 mg, twice daily, with meals.

- Vitamin C, 250 mg, twice daily, with the iron supplement (to increase iron absorption).

- Recommended increase in iron intake, including: organic, grass-fed red meat; organic beef or chicken liver; clams, oysters, mussels, and sardines; spinach, beans, and lentils paired with vitamin C–rich foods like bell peppers.

After two months, Kristen's iron markers had started to rise into the normal range. Simultaneously, her depressive symptoms lessened to the point where she returned to work, and she felt she was performing well. She was also sleeping through the night and felt energetic during the day, without needing to drink excessive amounts of caffeine (which she had been doing, to keep herself going). She also told me that she felt motivated to exercise and to seek out friends.

I recommended Kristen stay on iron and vitamin C, but at a reduced level of iron: 27 mg of iron bisglycinate once daily, with a meal; and 250 mg of vitamin C, once daily. She readily agreed—and continues to live and work without severe depression.

STEP-BY-STEP ACTION PLAN FOR

Minerals

Use this practical, step-by-step summary to implement the therapeutic actions discussed in this chapter.

Zinc

Step #1: If you're depressed, take zinc. I recommend 60 mg of zinc per day, 30 mg twice daily, with meals. (Zinc supplements can cause gastrointestinal upset if taken on an empty stomach.)

Caution: Zinc can deplete copper levels if you take more than 40 mg per day over a long period. A doctor should monitor your copper levels if you plan to take 60 mg or more long-term.

Step #2: Once you're in remission, take 30 mg per day, 15 mg two times daily, with meals.

Step #3: Eat more zinc-rich foods. They include oysters, red meat, eggs, wheat germ, spinach, pumpkin and squash seeds, nuts, chocolate, chicken, beans, and mushrooms.

Copper

Step #1: There are two ways to know for certain that you have excess copper and low zinc, a setup for depression: test for plasma copper and zinc levels; the Trace Mineral Hair Analysis, a hair test that measures zinc and copper levels.

Step #2: With results in hand, your doctor can definitively determine whether or not you have excess copper and low zinc. If you do, there's a straightforward, simple way to treat the problem: take zinc, at the doses specified in the "Zinc" section of this plan.

Step #3: If you're taking more than 40 mg of zinc per day, or if you have celiac disease or inflammatory bowel disease, ask your doctor to test you for low levels of copper.

Magnesium

Step #1: For a definitive analysis, consider testing for low magnesium. In my clinical experience, trace mineral analysis provides a simple, affordable, and useful tool for identifying magnesium deficiency.

Step #2: Talk to your doctor about clinical indicators of magnesium deficiency. They include anxiety, insomnia, constipation, and health conditions that involve muscle spasms (asthma, muscle cramps, migraines, eye twitching, etc.).

Step #3: Irrespective of testing or symptoms—take magnesium. Even without testing, I recommend a magnesium supplement for *every* patient with depression—because deficiency is so prevalent; and because magnesium is so safe and effective.

I typically recommend a dose of 240 mg, twice per day, either in the form of magnesium glycinate or magnesium citrate. (Magnesium oxide is poorly absorbed.) If you take magnesium threonate, the dose is 1,000 mg (which delivers 72 mg of elemental magnesium), twice per day. I recommend magnesium glycinate.

Step #4: Consider the form of magnesium you're taking. Some health experts recommend magnesium L-threonate as the best form of magnesium for the brain. That's because a few studies show brain-based benefits, like healthier brain cells and protection against age-related mental decline. There's nothing wrong with magnesium L-threonate, but it is more expensive than the other forms.

Some people *may* respond better to one form of magnesium versus another, so it can be worthwhile to switch forms to maximize benefits.

Caution: The main side effect from taking magnesium is loose stools. This laxative effect is most common with magnesium oxide, another reason not to use it. If you develop loose stools, split or decrease the dose, or switch to a slowly absorbed, long-acting form of magnesium.

Step #5: Eat more magnesium-rich foods. Magnesium supplements are a must for treating depression. But don't forget about increasing magnesium in your diet, too. The best sources are spinach and other dark green leafy vegetables, potatoes, beans, nuts and seeds, yogurt, oatmeal, brown rice, avocados, halibut, and wheat bran.

Chromium

Step #1: If you have the following disorders, diseases, or lifestyle factors, consider supplementing with chromium:

- atypical depression, with overeating and weight gain

- SAD

- PMDD

- prediabetes or diabetes

- overweight or obesity

- carbohydrate cravings

- seniors

Step #2: I recommend the supplement Trace Minerals, from Pure Encapsulations, which delivers 200 mcg per day of chromium, usually enough to restore normal levels and reduce or eliminate depressive symptoms.

Iron

Step #1: Get tested for levels of iron (particularly if you're a woman with heavy menstrual bleeding).

Step #2: If levels are low, eat more iron-rich foods (meat, poultry, seafood, beans, and iron-fortified cereals) and take iron-enhancing supplements.

Dose: 28 mg daily of *ferrous bisglycinate*, which doesn't cause the typical side effects of iron supplementation, like constipation, nausea, and stomach upset.

Goal: Iron levels higher than 50 g/dL, and ferritin levels close to 100 g/L.

Step #3: Take 250 mg of vitamin C with your iron supplement, to boost absorption.

Step #4: Retest after three months of supplementation. Once iron levels have normalized, you can stop taking the supplement.

Iodine

Step #1: If you want to include iodine in your Functional Psychiatry Treatment Plan, I recommend using the supplement Trace Minerals, from Pure Encapsulations, which delivers 100 mcg daily.

CHAPTER 8

Low-Dose Nutritional Lithium

Lowering the Risk of Suicide, Worldwide

> This unique mineral has the power to treat depression and reduce suicidality.

Lithium is an unusual mineral, so soft you can cut it with a knife, and so light it floats on water. In fact, it's often found in drinking water and soil—with studies from around the United States and worldwide linking low levels in an area's water supply to higher rates of mental and emotional disorders and violent crime. Let's explore together the way that lithium can help *your* mental health.

A History of Mental Healing

Back in the 1920s, the link between lithium and mood was so well known that a soft drink entrepreneur introduced a soda called Bib-Label Lithiated Lemon-Lime Soda with a slogan that promised an end to the inner pain of irritability and anger: "It takes the ouch out of the grouch." The soda was soon renamed 7UP. The "7" represented the rounded-up atomic weight of the element lithium (6.9). The "UP" pointed to the soda's ability to brighten mood. But don't look to today's 7UP to supply lithium—as of 1950, lithium citrate was no longer added as an ingredient to the soda.

Strange as it may seem, the original 7UP was part of an ancient medicinal tradition: people have been making use of the brain-balancing power of lithium for millennia.

Soranus, a physician in ancient Greece, prescribed "natural waters, such as alkaline springs" for people suffering manic episodes—springs we moderns have discovered are rich in lithium.

Lithia Springs, in Georgia, was the site of an ancient stone temple and an enormous earthen pyramid, both estimated to be thousands of years old. Later, it was a sacred healing site of the Cherokee. In 1888, Lithia Springs became a posh spa, subsequently used by American presidents like Cleveland, Taft, McKinley, and Theodore Roosevelt. Lithium-rich waters bottled at the spa—Bowden Lithia Water, delivering about 0.5 milligrams (mg) of lithium per liter—were sold widely in the United States and around the world from the 1880s to the end of World War I. At that time, medications containing lithium were also all the rage: by 1907, one medical textbook included forty-three different medicinal preparations containing the mineral.

After World War I, lithium's popularity faded. But in 1949, Australian physician John Cade used high doses of the mineral to treat "mania." By the 1970s, high-dose, pharmaceutical lithium had been approved by the FDA for "acute mania" and "recurrent" mania, and it became the standard treatment for manic depression. In the 1990s, however, there were new medications to treat "bipolar disorder" (a term first used in 1980, sparing people with the condition from being called "maniacs"), and pharmaceutical lithium became an afterthought. But that doesn't mean lithium itself has lost its therapeutic power or promise. Just the opposite.

How I Started Treating with Nutritional Lithium

In my opinion as a clinician, it's time for low-dose nutritional lithium to be included among nondrug treatments for emotional, mental, and behavioral disorders. (You can also find nutritional lithium in drinking water and in foods like vegetables, grains, meat, and fish. Also, many herbal experts say the spice thyme is rich in the mineral. However, you can't reliably get enough day-to-day nutritional lithium to make a symptom-relieving difference.) Nutritional lithium is certainly at the forefront of my psychiatry practice. I'd like to tell you the story of how I first started using the mineral—a story of bipolar disorder patients whose everyday lives were restored by the mineral.

High-dose pharmaceutical lithium (in the form of lithium carbonate) is an effective treatment for bipolar disorder, recurrent depression, and suicidal tendencies. But many physicians don't prescribe pharmaceutical lithium because of its potential to cause negative side effects, like irreversible kidney damage, thyroid disease, tremors, muscle weakness, poor coordination, tinnitus, and blurred vision.

In 1990, I was as familiar as any psychiatrist with these side effects. And I was also weary of constantly monitoring blood lithium levels in patients taking the drug to make sure levels were in the "therapeutic range"—a nonstop process that tends to shift the focus from the well-being of the patient to correct numbers from the lab. I started to wonder if *lower* doses of lithium might alleviate my patients' symptoms—without side effects.

I was led to low-dose lithium by Jonathan Wright, MD, a Harvard-trained physician who specializes in integrative medicine and nutritional therapies, and who had been treating people with low-dose nutritional lithium—and writing about it—for more than thirty years.

Like Dr. Wright, I began to prescribe the mineral in the form of lithium orotate or citrate, in low nutritional doses—doses far too low to generate the "therapeutic blood levels" of pharmaceutical lithium that require monitoring. To my delight, low-dose nutritional lithium had dramatic effects on mood and behavior in many patients.

Like Alice, a bipolar patient who was experiencing intolerable side effects from high-dose pharmaceutical lithium—and whose mood stabilized on a daily dose of 10 mg of nutritional lithium.

Or Pete, a fifty-year-old with severe bipolar disorder who developed chronic kidney disease on high-dose pharmaceutical lithium. Needless to say, he had to stop using the drug before it killed him. He was depressed and unemployed for three years—until he started taking 20 mg of nutritional lithium daily. In just a few weeks, he resumed everyday activities and returned to work.

Twenty-five years later, I continue to prescribe low-dose nutritional lithium to my patients. I use the treatment to stabilize mood, to help with addictions, to calm irritation and anger, to slow or stop memory loss in seniors. And to reverse depression—and the suicidality that is the most ominous symptom of depression.

Lowering Rates of Suicide Around the World

Lithium has been proven to have robust anti-suicide properties, not only in depressed and bipolar patients, but in the general public. An overwhelming body of evidence confirms this: not only are rates of suicide substantially lower among populations of lithium-treated bipolar patients, but rates of suicide are also lower in regions of the world where natural lithium exposures through drinking water are higher. In other words, where *more* lithium is present in groundwater and the food chain, rates of suicide and overall mortality are *lower*, often significantly.

For example, a 2020 study from Australian researchers analyzed data from twenty-seven other studies involving 113 million people—and found a link between higher lithium concentrations in drinking water and lower suicide rates, and between higher concentrations and lower rates of hospital admissions for psychiatric disorders like depression.[1]

Like many of the minerals discussed in this book, lithium probably works by affecting the serotonin pathway—with lithium helping the brain make more, store more, break down less, and release more serotonin. But lithium helps balance the brain in other ways. Lithium:

- inhibits glycogen synthase kinase 3 (GSK-3), preventing a cascade of neuroinflammation;

- increases the synthesis and action of brain-derived neurotrophic factor (BDNF), which supports the growth and maturation of brain cells;

Depression, Alzheimer's Disease— and Lithium

There is a well-proven link between depression and Alzheimer's disease. For example:

A study from Swedish researchers, published in 2023 in *Alzheimer's Research & Therapy*, analyzed health data from more than 1.3 million people. Those with a history of chronic or recurrent depression in midlife had more than double the risk of developing Alzheimer's—and those with a history of depression and chronic stress had four times the risk.[2]

The link seems clearly brain based. Both depression and Alzheimer's imbalance brain regions like the hippocampus, amygdala, and prefrontal cortex, which regulate mood, memory, and cognition. Both are marked by neuroinflammation. In some cases, depression in older adults may even be an early sign of Alzheimer's disease.

All the more reason to take supplemental low-dose nutritional lithium if you're depressed! Consider this evidence.

Seven times lower risk. In a study published in the *British Journal of Psychiatry*, researchers found that bipolar patients treated with lithium had a *seven times* lower rate of developing Alzheimer's than bipolar patients taking other medications.[3]

Sixteen thousand patients provide more proof. In research published in the *Archives of General Psychiatry*, Danish scientists analyzed data from more than sixteen thousand psychiatric patients who had used lithium, and found they had a low rate of Alzheimer's and other types of dementia.[4]

Fifty-nine percent less risk. In a meta-analysis of seven studies on lithium and dementia, published in *European Neurology* in 2024, lithium therapy reduced the risk of Alzheimer's disease by 59 percent, and the risk of any kind of dementia by 66 percent.[5]

The potential to prevent Alzheimer's. Brazilian researchers studied forty-five people with mild cognitive impairment (MCI), a form of mental decline that can lead to Alzheimer's. (Ten to 15 percent of people with MCI develop Alzheimer's.) Over twelve months, half of them took low-dose lithium and half took a placebo. At the end of the study, those on lithium had: decreased levels of tau, the "tangles" in neurons linked to Alzheimer's (the placebo group had higher levels); improved performance on a test measuring the cognitive factors of Alzheimer's disease; and better focus and stronger memory. Lithium, concluded the researchers in the *British Journal of Psychiatry*, has the potential to prevent Alzheimer's disease.[6] A subsequent two-year study by the same team of researchers, involving sixty-one older people with MCI, produced similar results: those receiving the placebo had cognitive and functional decline, while those taking lithium remained stable—and even experienced improvements in memory and focus.[7]

More lithium in the water, less dementia. In a study published in 2017 in *JAMA Psychiatry*, Danish researchers analyzed data on lithium and dementia from more than 800,000 people. They found that people with higher levels of lithium in their drinking water had a 17 percent lower risk of dementia and Alzheimer's disease. "Increased lithium exposure in drinking water may be associated with a lower incidence of dementia," the researchers concluded.[8]

And in a similar study published in 2018 in the *Journal of Alzheimer's Disease*, higher levels of lithium in drinking water in Texas were linked to lower rates of death from Alzheimer's disease (and deaths from obesity and type 2 diabetes).[9]

Bottom line: If you're depressed, you're at increased risk for Alzheimer's disease and other forms of dementia. Low-dose nutritional lithium lowers your risk.

- is anti-inflammatory, protecting against neuroinflammation; and

- increases brain volume in areas that process emotion and thinking.

All those neuroprotective actions make a real difference—in fact, a remarkable difference. Research shows that low-dose lithium can slow *mild cognitive impairment* (the mental decline that can lead to Alzheimer's disease) and stabilize Alzheimer's. Studies also show low-dose lithium can aid in the treatment of addiction and substance use disorders.

There is also research showing low-dose nutritional lithium can help with depression.

A study published in the *Journal of the American Association of Nurse Practitioners* in 2024 found that low-dose lithium reduced symptoms of depression by 66 percent and anxiety by 65 percent in people with major depression, bipolar disorder, and generalized anxiety disorder.[10]

A study published in the *Neuroscience and Biobehavioral Reviews* in 2023 reported that low-dose lithium reduced depressive symptoms in adults with mild cognitive impairment.[11]

And low-dose nutritional lithium is particularly effective at treating people who are depressed *and* angry.

Irritability and Anger: Two Overlooked Symptoms of Depression

The DSM-5-TR—the *Diagnostic and Statistical Manual of Mental Disorders, Fifth Edition* (Text Revision)—is the authoritative text used by psychiatrists, psychologists, and other mental health professionals to diagnose and classify mental health disorders. And in the DSM-5-TR, *irritability* is recognized as a possible symptom of depression in children and adolescents—but not in adults.

Personally, I think that's a mistake. In my clinical experience, many depressed or bipolar adults are also irritable and angry—sometimes even full of rage, and aggressive. This irritability is often one factor in a particular pattern that indicates an individual may derive a *lot* of benefit from the brain-balancing, calming effect of lithium. The pattern looks like this:

- A previous or current psychiatric diagnosis, especially depression, bipolar disorder, or borderline personality disorder

- Symptoms like irritability, anger, hostility, anxiety, mood swings, compulsive behavior, or a history of self-injury

- Past or current substance abuse

- Suicidality

- A family history of any of the above

Allen is a very good example of someone who fit the above pattern. Here's his remarkable story of rage—and lithium-aided relief.

Allen did not come in for treatment willingly. I had been treating Allen's stepson for ADHD when his wife, Samantha, approached me with her concerns about Allen. She described the following incident to explain Allen's typical behavior:

"We were driving to my parents' house for dinner one Sunday when another driver cut in front of us. Allen began to curse and honk his horn excessively until the driver pulled over, allowing Allen to pass. Instead of driving away, Allen's anger continued to escalate until he got out of his truck, grabbed a crowbar from the trunk, and started charging toward the other driver. The driver sped off and fortunately nobody was hurt, but at that point I knew that Allen needed help."

Allen did not believe he had an anger problem. He had been on several antidepressant medications in the past to control his mood, including Zoloft and Prozac. While these medications seemed to be effective in helping Allen control his depression, his uncontrolled levels of irritability remained.

After several repeated attempts, Samantha finally got Allen to seek help. When he arrived at my office for his scheduled appointment, he proceeded to scream at my administrative assistant for "making" him fill out "so many stupid" forms. To make matters worse, I was running fifteen minutes behind schedule, which only intensified his anger.

Allen entered my office in the same belligerent state; he glared at me and shouted several expletives seemingly directed at no one in particular. Eventually, he was able to discuss his ongoing issues with anger but remained hostile throughout our session.

During my initial visit with Allen, I learned that he had lost several jobs earlier in his life and had a history of alcoholism, depression, and irritability. When asked about his family, he reported that his father and many uncles were alcoholics. He had left his childhood home at the age of eighteen and was not close with his family. At this time, however, Allen had been sober for more than ten years, and functioned in a high-level sales job.

After Allen settled down and I was able to ask more detailed questions about his childhood, medical history, family history, and past attempts of therapy and medications, I realized that he was caught in a mental health system that couldn't adequately treat his problem.

Allen went to therapy as a teenager and had been on and off antidepressants since the age of sixteen. When the irritability persisted, even after therapy and multiple medications, he found success in Alcoholics Anonymous (AA), which helped him quit drinking, but didn't address his underlying irritability and anger. Allen had never hurt anyone, but he had experienced "road rage" for years. Incidents like the one his partner Samantha described had been a consistent feature of Allen's life. I recommended he take 5 mg of nutritional lithium daily for a month, and we scheduled a follow-up session.

When I met Allen for the second time approximately one month after our initial meeting, he came to the office with Samantha. Allen was calm and inquisitive about his lab tests. He reported no side effects on the 5 mg of lithium and described a week without any episodes of road rage.

His wife thought Allen was less irritable at home and had, as an example, tolerated a long wait in a restaurant where they had a reservation—typically, she explained, these were the kinds of incidents that sent him "over the edge."

During our second session, we mostly discussed the laboratory test that had detected low levels of vitamin D, and I prescribed 5,000 international units (IU) of vitamin D. I also asked Allen to increase his nutritional lithium to 10 mg twice a day.

When Allen returned for his second follow-up visit, after three months on the 10 mg of lithium and Vitamin D, he walked toward me, smiled, and shook my hand. The gratitude in his eyes was apparent. As we completed our session, he expressed his remorse over how his irritability and angry outbursts impacted his family and others.

Low-Dose Nutritional Lithium Is Safe

Before I discuss the protocol for supplementing with this mineral, I want to emphasize the *safety* of low-dose lithium orotate—since high-dose lithium carbonate can be so dangerous.

As a dietary supplement, lithium orotate has been marketed and utilized worldwide for decades—a real-world testament to its safety. And my clinical experience has shown me that low-dose nutritional lithium is very safe. But experts within the medical and scientific communities continue to raise concerns about its safety. I think there are a few reasons for those concerns: the serious side effects of pharmaceutical lithium; the narrow therapeutic window for pharmaceutical lithium; and the fact that, until recently, the research on lithium orotate has been quite sparse.

To address the gaps in research on lithium orotate, a team of scientists conducted a study to explore its "safety profile," looking at its potential toxicity to genes and toxicity from repeated oral doses. Their results were published in 2021 in *Regulatory Toxicology and Pharmacology*—and they were very reassuring. They found that lithium orotate did *not* cause genetic toxicity. And in a twenty-eight-day study on laboratory animals, they found that repeated high doses—400 mg per kilogram of body weight, per day—had no adverse effects. "These results are supportive of the history of use of lithium orotate without significant postmarket safety signal generation," wrote the researchers.[12] In plain English: the safety of lithium orotate has been proven in the marketplace, and now it's been proven in this study.

Finally Hopeful Success Story

PATIENT: Phoebe

TREATMENT FOR: Depression, alcoholism, anger, and irritability

Phoebe was a forty-three-year-old therapist who had been diagnosed with depression and alcohol abuse when she was eighteen. As I took her history, she told me her family had been deeply impaired by alcoholism—her parents, her siblings, and herself. She had been taking an antidepressant, and said she was working hard at maintaining her sobriety, which she had done for the past ten years. But she had come to me for additional support because she was afraid of a relapse, describing herself as a "dry drunk," desperately clinging to "white-knuckle sobriety." Last but not least, Phoebe told me she was chronically irritable—and prone to outbursts of anger at her family.

Phoebe had many of the signs of low lithium. Depression. Alcoholism, including a family history of alcoholism. Irritability and anger. And Trace Mineral Hair Analysis revealed a low level of the mineral.

I prescribed a daily dose of 5 mg of nutritional lithium, and scheduled a return visit in six weeks.

Once she had settled herself for our second visit, Phoebe burst into tears—of relief. For the first time in her life, she told me, she was *not* constantly irritable. And that change was a huge relief for her, even joyous.

She also expressed regret about her family having to tolerate her irritability and anger for so many years. I listened closely, and with respect. And then I told her that she had a nutritional imbalance—probably genetically inherited—that predisposed her to depression, anger, and irritability. She did not have a *behavioral* problem, per se. She had a *biological* problem that had been detected and treated. I counseled her to apologize to her family, forgive herself—and enjoy the rest of her calmer, more balanced life.

The Right Dose

For maximum safety, I start patients on a daily dose of 2 mg of lithium orotate. (I recommend the 1 mg product from Pure Encapsulations, taking 1 mg with breakfast and 1 with dinner.) That's a good level of supplementation for anyone who is depressed.

After two to four weeks, if there are no side effects, I may increase the dosage. For people with bipolar disorder and addiction, for example, I may gradually increase the dosage up to 20 or 30 mg daily, increasing by 5 mg every two weeks. For people with the anger-including depressive pattern I described earlier, I may increase the dosage up to 10 mg. For these regimens, I use the 5 mg product from Pure Encapsulations, in divided doses, with meals.

However, if you take *more* than 10 mg of lithium orotate, I strongly advise you to work with a functional doctor who understands how to utilize low-dose nutritional lithium; a doctor who can help you determine the most effective dose for *you*, and who can monitor you for any possible side effects.

One last precaution: There's not enough evidence to say that low-dose nutritional lithium is safe for pregnant women or women trying to conceive.

STEP-BY-STEP ACTION PLAN FOR

Low-Dose Nutritional Lithium

Use this practical, step-by-step summary to implement the therapeutic actions discussed in this chapter.

Step #1: Start taking 2 mg of lithium orotate. I recommend the 1 mg product from Pure Encapsulations, taking 1 mg with breakfast and 1 with dinner.

Step #2: After two to four weeks, if there are no side effects, increase the dosage to 5 mg, using the 5 mg product from Pure Encapsulations.

Step #3: For people with the anger-including depressive pattern described in this chapter, increase the dosage up to 10 mg. Again, use the 5 mg supplement, in divided doses, with meals.

   Cautions: If you take more than 10 mg of lithium orotate, work with a functional doctor who understands how to utilize low-dose nutritional lithium; a doctor who can help you determine the most effective dose for *you*, and who can monitor you for any possible side effects.

   If you're pregnant or trying to conceive, you shouldn't take low-dose nutritional lithium because there's not enough evidence to definitively say it is safe for you.

CHAPTER 9

Essential Fats, Essential Healing

Omega-3 fatty acids are a must for healthy neurons—and for your happiness.

As I wrote in my book *Finally Focused*, there's a reason why the American Psychiatric Association (APA) recommends that every man, woman, and child in America eat fish—particularly fatty fish like salmon and sardines—two or more times a week. And why the APA also recommends that people with mood disorders like depression supplement their daily diet with 1 or more grams (g) of a fish oil supplement.

The reason is—we're all fatheads. Literally.

Yes, 60 percent of your brain is *fat*—which means that your brain needs a steady supply of dietary fat for its health and well-being. Specifically, your brain depends on *essential fatty acids* (EFA), the building blocks of fat. (They're called "essential" because your body doesn't manufacture them—you have to get them from your diet.) And fatty fish and fish oil supply two of the most important EFAs for your brain: eicosapentaenoic acid (EPA); and docosahexaenoic acid (DHA).

Both of these fatty acids are *omega-3s*, a chemical label indicating the placement of double-bonded carbon atoms in a fat molecule. But fittingly, *omega* is also the Greek word for *great*—because when enough omega-3s are on the job, they do a great job protecting your brain. But if levels are low:

- the outer covering (membrane) of brain cells (neurons) degenerates;

- neurotransmitter signaling, which helps control mood, mental activity, and behavior, is disrupted;

- cellular receptors for the neurotransmitter *dopamine* become malformed, lowering dopamine levels—and low dopamine is a recognized cause of depression;

- there also are fewer *synapses*, the bridges between neurons; and

- neurons are more likely to atrophy in response to stress, anxiety, and depression.

In short, just about every aspect of *neurotransmission*—the movement of information from neuron to neuron that underlies every emotion, thought, and action—depends on omega-3s. Omega-3s also protect the brain by decreasing chronic low-grade inflammation, the chronic cellular fire that can singe neurons, and is an acknowledged cause of depression. (Some experts go so far as to say neuroinflammation is *the* cause of depression.)

Bottom line: A deficiency of omega-3s is bad news for your brain. And omega-3 deficiency is common.

Our hunter-gatherer ancestors ate a diet with a ratio of about two-to-one omega-6s to omega-3s. Omega-6s are another essential fatty acid (EFA), found mainly in meat, poultry, eggs, and nuts and seeds. There's nothing wrong with omega-6s—they're also a must for a healthy brain. But when the *balance* of omega-3s and omega-6s is skewed—when you're eating too many omega-6s and too few omega-3s—the body flips into a pro-inflammatory state. And that's exactly the composition of the American diet. In contrast to the balanced, healthy ratio of two-to-one, most Americans eat a diet with a ruinous ratio of fifteen-to-one. (In the modern diet, omega-6s are mostly from mass-produced meat, vegetable oils, and other processed foods.) This double whammy—a barrage of omega-6s and a paucity of omega-3s—is a little-recognized factor in the symptoms of depression.

Little recognized, that is, by doctors. But not by nutritional scientists. There have been more studies conducted on the link between depression and omega-3s than on any other nutrient. Let's take a look at some of that science.

A Fish Story You Can Believe

A "fish story" is the classic example of a fib—an angler exaggerating the size of their catch. But there's nothing exaggerated about the sizable effect of omega-3s on depression.

Ten studies tell the tale: EPA tames depression. In a study published in 2023, English researchers analyzed the results of ten other studies on EPA/DHA and depression, involving nearly 1,500 people. They found that 1 to 2 g per day of fish oil (60 percent EPA) led to a "significant reduction in depression severity."[1] In similar research, published in 2019, scientists analyzed the results of twenty-six studies on omega-3 and depression, involving more than two thousand people—and found that giving 60 percent EPA at a dosage of 1 g or less per day had "beneficial effects on depression."[2]

Less inflammation = less depression. Why is EPA the most effective fatty acid for treating depression? Probably because it's the most effective at reducing inflammation, according to a team of researchers from Tufts University, Emory University, and Harvard Medical School. The researchers studied forty-five people with major depressive disorder (MDD) and high levels of C-reactive protein (CRP), a biomarker for chronic inflammation. They divided them into four groups, with four different supplement regimens: 1, 2, or 4 g of omega-3 per day, or a placebo. (The omega-3 supplement had a ratio of four-to-one EPA to DHA.)

After three months of supplementation, the group getting 4 g had the best response, with two out of three participants in the group experiencing a 50 percent or greater reduction in depressive symptoms—meaning fish oil was nearly three times more powerful than the placebo.

The 4 g group also had much higher levels of *specialized pro-resolving mediators*, or SPMs—molecules derived from omega-3s that play a crucial role in cooling inflammation and repairing inflammation-caused damage.

They also had the biggest decrease in CRP.

This study "highlights the activation of the resolution of inflammation as a likely mechanism in the treatment of major depressive disorder with omega-3 fatty acid supplementation," wrote the researchers in the May 2023 issue of *Neuropsychopharmacology*.[3]

Less fish during pregnancy, more depression afterward. In a 2021 study, Japanese researchers looked at eighty pregnant women, tracking their fish consumption and blood levels of EPA. Those who ate less fish during pregnancy had lower levels of EPA—and a greater risk of postpartum depression (PD), a problem suffered by up to 16 percent of new mothers.[4]

High omega-6 and low omega-3 is a setup for depression. In a seven-year study from Australian researchers, people who had much higher levels of omega-6 than omega-3 in their cells were 89 percent more likely to develop a mood disorder like depression.[5]

Evidence you can salute. In a study published in *Military Medicine*, a psychiatrist and captain in the U.S. Public Health Service reviewed the many studies on omega-3 and depression. He found:

- when fish consumption decreases and omega-6 intake increases, the risk of depression goes up;

- higher tissue levels of EPA and DHA lower the risk of depression; and

- supplementing the diet with omega-3s—with a higher ratio of EPA than DHA—relieves depressive symptoms.

"Rebalancing of the essential fatty acid composition of U.S. military diets . . . may help reduce military psychiatric distress," he concluded.[6]

An earlier study, published in the *Journal of Clinical Psychiatry*, came to a similar conclusion: military personnel with low levels of omega-3s were 62 percent more likely to die from suicide compared to personnel with high levels.[7]

A risk factor in other types of mental decline. Depression isn't the only mental health problem caused or worsened by low blood levels of

What About Alpha-Linoleic Acid (ALA)?

There are three major types of essential omega-3 fatty acids: EPA and DHA, found mainly in seafood; and ALA, found mainly in plant foods like flaxseeds, chia seeds, and walnuts. While the body can convert ALA to EPA and DHA, the conversion is *slow*. And it depends on other nutritional factors, like zinc. That's why I favor *direct consumption* of EPA and DHA—through supplements and seafood—as the best way to normalize blood levels.

omega-3s. A study by European researchers analyzed results from thirty-six studies looking at the link between omega-3s and mental health. They found low levels were a risk factor not only for major depression and PD, but also for psychosis and dementia. The results were published in 2023 in *Frontiers in Psychiatry*.[8]

The Best Dose

To treat depression, consider taking up to 3 g of fish oil per day, with an EPA to DHA ratio of three-to-one.

Think twice about the supplement you're taking. The ocean is polluted with mercury, cadmium, arsenic, and other heavy metals, and they "bioaccumulate" in fish. Other toxic chemicals—like polychlorinated biphenyls (PCBs), polybrominated biphenyls (PBBs), dioxins, and furans—can also build up in the tissues and organs of fish, and end up in your tissues and organs when you take a fish oil supplement.

So make sure your fish oil (or krill oil, or algae) omega-3 supplement is from a company that adheres to stringent standards for product testing and purity.

(EPA- and DHA-containing algae supplements are a good option for vegetarians.)

But here's the good news about fish oil and pollutants.

In a test from consumerlab.com, thirty-three fish oil supplements passed with flying colors, with no contamination from mercury and very little residues of PCBs.

The supplement I recommend for my patients: Equazen, which is specifically formulated to support brain function, providing an ideal balance of omega-3s *and* omega-6 (www.equazen.com).

You can also boost omega-3s with diet.

Eat seafood at least twice a week, especially wild-caught salmon, sardines, and herring. Grill or bake the fish. Try to avoid farmed fish, which may be high in mercury and other contaminants.

Eat meats like beef, pork, and lamb from grass-fed animals, which contain a higher omega-3 to omega-6 ratio.

Plant foods that deliver a goodly amount of omega-3s include flaxseeds and flaxseed oil, chia seeds, walnuts, pecans, pumpkin seeds, sesame seeds, tahini, hummus, tofu, and fresh spinach. But don't count on plant foods to deliver all the omega-3s you need.

Finally Hopeful Success Story

PATIENT: Tracy
TREATMENT FOR: MDD, cutting, ADHD

Tracy, a fifteen-year-old girl, came to my office in September with her mother, Joanne, who said she had a history of "spacy" behavior and an annoying predilection to imitate her family and friends. During the visit, Joanne shared her concerns about Tracy's eating habits and recent weight gain. She said she had found hidden candy wrappers around the house—in the back of drawers, under rugs, in the cracks of the couch in the living room. Over the summer, Joanne told me, Tracy had gained twenty-five pounds.

More worrying was the fact that Tracy had consistently worn long-sleeved clothing during the hot days of summer. When confronted by her parents, Tracy revealed that she had been cutting her arms to relieve stress. At that point, her parents scheduled an appointment with me.

During my conversation with Tracy, she told me she felt depressed. Her primary care doctor had prescribed two antidepressant medications, Prozac (fluoxetine) and Lexapro (escitalopram). But Prozac had triggered thoughts of suicide, and Lexapro had caused severe nausea. Tracy stopped using both.

My physical exam showed that Tracy had two skin conditions: eczema; and keratosis pilaris, small, rough, and red bumps on her upper arms and neck.

Both of these conditions are telltale signs of the need for more of the essential fatty acids (EFAs): EPA, DHA, and gamma-linolenic acid (GLA). Tracy didn't meet diagnostic criteria for binge eating disorder, but she was clearly struggling with binging on sweets.

Based on her medical history and physical exam, I ordered laboratory testing to identify underlying factors that could be contributing to her symptoms.

And, in fact, the laboratory results showed that the levels of EPA, DHA, and GLA in her blood cells were very low. She also had low levels of the mineral magnesium.

My diagnosis: major depressive disorder; eating disorder, not otherwise specified; EFA deficiency; and magnesium deficiency.

The Functional Psychiatry Treatment Plan for Tracy:

EFA supplement of 2 g of combined EPA/DHA/GLA, twice daily. As discussed in this chapter, omega-3 fatty acids are critical for normal brain function, with a 2024 study from Chinese and Canadian researchers showing that in children and adolescents a combination of EFAs and therapy had a 92 percent success rate in clearing up depression. Other research shows that GLA levels are low in people with depression—just as they were in Tracy.

Magnesium glycinate, 240 mg, twice daily. As discussed in Chapter 7, magnesium plays many roles in brain health, and has proven effective in treating depression.   *(continued)*

One month later: no more cutting

Tracy and her parents were back in my office four weeks later. Her parents said they noted some small improvements in Tracy's behavior. Tracy said that she was in a much better mood—and she'd stopped cutting to deal with stress.

During this visit, Tracy's parents told me about a previous diagnosis they'd failed to mention in the initial visit: attention-deficit/hyperactivity disorder (ADHD). Tracy had been diagnosed with ADHD when she was eight but never received any treatment. When I talked to her, Tracy said she struggled to focus on activities both at school and at home and was often reprimanded for not paying attention. Based on this additional info, I expanded Tracy's treatment to address all her symptoms, adding 30 mg a day of the ADHD stimulant drug Vyvanse (lisdexamfetamine), and a recommendation for therapy for Tracy and her family.

Four months later: major improvement

When I saw Tracy and her parents four months later, Tracy was markedly improved. Her school performance was being praised by her teachers, and she was no longer being reprimanded. Her homelife was more stable, with Tracy's parents feeling like therapy had provided significant insights about Tracy.

And testing showed that Tracy's levels of EFAs had normalized. Over the next few months, we were able to slowly reduce and then eliminate the ADHD medication, without any return of ADHD symptoms.

Tracy's case illustrates a fundamental feature of Functional and Integrative Psychiatry: it uses *all* the tools available for healing. In this case, those were: laboratory testing; targeted nutritional supplementation; medications; and therapy.

Essential Testing

How can you make sure you've got plenty of omega-3 on board?

There are many different tests to measure blood levels of EFAs, from many different labs, like Genova Diagnostics and Quest Diagnostics. (There are also omega-3 tests you can order directly, like the Omega Index from OmegaQuant.) But since deficiency of omega-3s is so common, I think taking up to 3 g of omega-3 per day for three months without testing is safe and sensible. After three months, get tested. If your ratio of omega-6s to omega-3s is not two-to-one, increase your dose of omega-3s.

However, don't expect results overnight from omega-3 supplementation. It takes time to "change the oil" in your body. In fact, if you have a chronic deficiency, it can take up to ten weeks to achieve healthy omega-3 levels through supplementation.

The Cholesterol Connection

There's another fat I'd like to discuss in this chapter. It's not considered an essential fat like omega-3s. But it's so important to health that your body manufactures it. And for a sizable number of people, having normal blood levels is a must for healing depression. I'm talking about *cholesterol.*

Cholesterol? Surprising, right? You know cholesterol as a blood fat that's linked to cardiovascular disease, like the "bad" low-density lipoprotein (LDL) cholesterol that raises the risk of heart attack and stroke, and the "good" high-density lipoprotein (HDL) cholesterol that lowers risk. But cholesterol is much, much more.

This waxy substance is vital for the production of hormones like estrogen and testosterone. It's also an indispensable ingredient of cell membranes—and deficiency makes it more difficult to transmit signals from cell to cell. Cholesterol provides a protective coating for nerve cells. And without cholesterol, you can't make vitamin D, which itself is cru-

Finally Hopeful Success Story

PATIENT: Ted, a seventeen-year-old
TREATED FOR: Depression, addiction, and self-harm

Ted was seventeen when he and his family came to my office, asking for help. Ted had been struggling with severe depression for years. He had developed self-harming behaviors as a coping mechanism, often cutting his forearms and thighs with a razor, much to the concern of his parents. Ted also struggled with addiction to cannabis and benzodiazepines, crushing and snorting Xanax tablets that had been prescribed for his father.

Ted's family history included depression in his mother and sister, while his father struggled with panic attacks. The family had limited funds, so laboratory testing consisted of tests fully covered by insurance.

My initial testing revealed two very relevant findings: a very low total cholesterol level of 92 milligrams per deciliter (mg/dL), along with vitamin D deficiency. As I explain in this chapter, low total cholesterol levels are linked to depression, suicide, self-harming, and addiction. Similarly, low vitamin D levels are linked to suicidal behaviors and addiction, and vitamin D has proven itself useful in the treatment of depression.

For Ted, the Functional Psychiatry Treatment Plan consisted of:

- Sonic Cholesterol (a cholesterol supplement), two tabs, three times per day;
- vitamin D3, 10,000 international units (IU) per day; and
- Creon (pancrelipase, a prescription digestive enzyme, to help with cholesterol digestion), with meals and snacks.

Two months: the first signs of improvement

At the two-month follow-up, Ted had reduced cutting behaviors and was actively pursuing outpatient addiction treatment. He was also talking about attending college, a first for him.

My follow-up testing showed a slight boost in total cholesterol to 100 mg/dL—but that wasn't bad news. Targeted nutritional supplementation with cholesterol usually increases blood levels of total cholesterol slowly, and often by only small amounts. The goal is not a certain level of total cholesterol; it's symptom improvement—and that's what was happening with Ted. He also had a normalization of his vitamin D levels, at 33 nanograms per milliliter (ng/mL). I continued Ted on the same dose of Sonic Cholesterol, changed his daily vitamin D supplement to 5,000 IU, and continued with the Creon.

I saw Ted about twice a year over the next few years. While he still struggled with some depressive symptoms, he no longer had severe depression. He was *motivated*, pursuing realistic goals for his future. He signed up for classes at the local community college, and started working toward a degree. He stayed sober. And after he graduated from community college—a very happy day for Ted and his parents—he started attending university.

cial to brain functioning (as you read about in Chapter 5). In fact, the brain is the most cholesterol-rich organ in the body.

Cholesterol is so important to health and well-being that most of it— 85 percent—is manufactured in the body, in the liver and other organs. Only 15 percent comes from food.

Cholesterol can be a health hero. But, of course, the conversation about cholesterol is often only about the damage done by high levels, with the emphasis on *lowering* total and LDL cholesterol to prevent heart disease. For some people, however, that's a big mistake—a mistake that can lead to depression. Research links low levels of total cholesterol to depression. For example:

Three times the risk of depression. A 1993 paper published in the *Lancet* reported, "Among men aged seventy years and older, categorically defined depression was three times more common in the group with low total plasma cholesterol . . . than in those with higher concentrations."[9]

Long-term low cholesterol, more depressive symptoms. In a 2000 study published in *Psychosomatic Medicine*, researchers compared cholesterol levels to depressive symptoms in men aged forty to seventy. They found that men with long-term, low total cholesterol levels "have a higher prevalence of depressive symptoms" compared to those with higher cholesterol levels.[10]

True for women, too. Women with low cholesterol levels are also vulnerable to depression. In 1998, Swedish researchers reported the results of their examination of cholesterol and depressive symptoms among three hundred healthy women, ages thirty-one to sixty-five. Women with the lowest levels of cholesterol suffered from significantly more depressive symptoms than did the others.[11]

Results from Italy and Ireland. Italian researchers measured the cholesterol levels of 186 patients hospitalized for depression and found an association between low cholesterol and depressive symptoms.[12]

In a similar study, published in 2001 in *Psychiatry Research*, primary care patients in Ireland with low levels of cholesterol had higher ratings on depression rating scales.[13]

More evidence from a meta-analysis. In a 2008 meta-analysis, higher total cholesterol was associated with lower levels of depression.[14]

Low HDL, more symptoms. A 2010 study published in the *Journal of Neuropsychiatry & Clinical Neurosciences* looked at the levels of HDL in depressed people and found that low levels of HDL were linked to "long-term depressive symptomatology."[15]

High cholesterol, fewer suicidal thoughts. Croatian scientists studied 203 men with PTSD, looking at depression, aggression, suicidality—and cholesterol. They found that the men with the highest cholesterol levels had less risk of suicidal ideation (thinking about committing suicide); less risk of significant aggression; and fewer depressive symptoms.[16]

Low HDL, more severe fatigue. In a 2024 study published in the *Journal of Psychosomatic Research*, psychiatrists from Taiwan found that people with MDD were three times more likely to suffer from severe fatigue if their HDL cholesterol level was low.[17]

Other research links low cholesterol to eating disorders; substance abuse and relapse; self-injury; lack of impulse control; and even homicide.

Another cholesterol connection: cholesterol-lowering statin drugs are taken by 25 percent of American adults—and they're linked to a range of psychiatric effects, including depression, suicidality (thinking about, attempting, or committing suicide), anxiety, nightmares, irritability, and aggression.

Yet another connection: antidepressant medications may further lower cholesterol, counteracting any potential benefit.

My clinical experience and conclusion: Cholesterol levels and family history are highly predictive of mental health risk. A family history of aggression, violence, substance abuse, and/or suicidality may indicate an inherited metabolic defect that interferes with the normal synthesis and recycling of serum cholesterol—and a need for greater intake.

Bottom line: If you're depressed, or experience suicidality (a form of violence, against yourself), or have the family history I just described—you should have your cholesterol levels checked.

If your level of total cholesterol is *below* 140 mg/dL, I advise pushing it back up *above* 160.

For some people, that means working with their doctor to decrease the dosage of cholesterol-lowering medication, allowing levels to rise naturally. For people with moderately low cholesterol—110 to 160—a cholesterol-rich diet can help. That means eating several servings a week of eggs and other cholesterol-rich foods, like full-fat dairy products. For eggs, I favor eating organic, free-range eggs, one of the richest sources of dietary cholesterol. Eggs also supply healthy amounts of protein, B vitamins, choline, and other brain-supporting nutrients. In my view, eggs and dairy are healthy foods, and there's no reason to be afraid of them. One caveat: Don't consume these foods if you're sensitive or allergic to them—about one in twenty people for dairy, and one in two hundred for eggs.

If your total cholesterol is under 110, you should consider taking a *cholesterol supplement* to raise levels. Dietary changes alone won't make a significant difference. (Remember, 85 percent of the cholesterol in the body is made in the liver, with only 15 percent from the diet. So, dietary changes can get you only so far.)

I favor Sonic Cholesterol, the prescription cholesterol supplement from New Beginnings Nutritionals. Your doctor can order the supplement at www.nbnus.net. Or, you can write New Beginnings Nutritionals at info@nbnus.com, and they will recommend a medical practitioner who can work with you via telemedicine to prescribe the supplement.

Here are the dosages for this supplement:

For very low cholesterol values (< 100 mg/dl or 2.59 millimoles per liter—mmol/L): Dose 4–6 capsules (1,000–1,500 mg) per day in divided doses with meals.

For moderately low cholesterol values (100 to 130 mg/dl or 2.59 to 3.36 mmol/L): Dose 3–4 capsules (750–1,000 mg) per day in divided doses with meals.

Precautions: I strongly recommend quarterly cholesterol testing for a time to monitor and adjust cholesterol dosing until blood levels are stabilized. After levels are stabilized, I recommend testing every six months.

Along with this supplement, consider taking bile acids, a compound generated in the liver that helps digest fat. Also consider taking a supplement containing lipase, a type of digestive enzyme that helps break down fat. The supplement Digestion GB, from Pure Encapsulation, delivers both bile acids and lipase.

One last point: When I suspect low cholesterol in depression, I also order a test for pregnenolone, a mood-supporting hormone made from cholesterol. You can read more about pregnenolone in Chapter 12.

EFAs

Use this practical, step-by-step summary to implement the therapeutic actions discussed in this chapter.

EFAs

Step #1: To treat depression, take up to 3 g of fish oil per day, with an EPA to DHA ratio of three-to-one. I favor the supplement Equazen, which provides an ideal ratio of omega-3s and omega-6s. Testing is not necessary before starting supplementation.

Step #2: After three months of supplementation, test for omega-3 levels, and work with your doctor to adjust supplementation accordingly. Ongoing, test every six months to ensure levels are normal.

Step #3: Maximize omega-3s in your diet. Eat seafood at least twice a week, especially salmon, sardines, albacore tuna (low in mercury), mackerel, and herring. Eat meats from grass-fed animals. Eat plant foods that deliver omega-3s, including flaxseeds and flaxseed oil, chia seeds, walnuts, pecans, pumpkin seeds, tahini, hummus, tofu, and fresh spinach.

Cholesterol

Step #1: If you're depressed or experiencing suicidality (thinking about or attempting suicide), have your total cholesterol checked. If it is below 160 mg/dL, consider a prescription cholesterol supplement—I recommend Sonic Cholesterol, from New Beginnings Nutritionals—and use according to the dosage recommendations in the chapter.

Step #2: If cholesterol is below 160, consider eating more cholesterol-rich foods, like eggs and full-fat dairy products.

Step #3: If cholesterol is below 160, work with your doctor to adjust your cholesterol-lowering medication.

Step #4: I strongly recommend quarterly cholesterol testing for a time to monitor and adjust cholesterol dosing until blood levels are stabilized. After levels are stabilized, I recommend testing every six months.

Step #5: Take a supplement containing bile acids and lipases, both of which help digest fat. I recommend Digestion GB, from Pure Encapsulations.

Step #6: Also test for pregnenolone, a mood-balancing hormone made from cholesterol. (Therapeutic actions for pregnenolone are discussed in Chapter 12.)

CHAPTER 10

Polyphenols

Powerful Phytochemicals in Plants and Foods

> Natural chemicals can do
> wonders for your mood.

When you're depressed, your life is drained of color.

Well, it's time to put color back into your life—specifically, the *red* in red grapes, the *blue* in blueberries, the *green* in green tea, and the *deep brown* in pine bark.

All of these botanicals are rich in oligomeric proanthocyanidins (OPCs), a type of polyphenol, a compound that plants produce to protect themselves from environmental harm.

Often, the polyphenol is a plant pigment, which acts like a natural sunscreen, protecting plants from the sun's unrelenting ultraviolet radiation. These pigments are also loaded with antioxidants, which cut down on cell-damaging oxidation. (When you slice an apple, exposing its delicate flesh to the air, and it immediately browns—that's oxidation.)

But polyphenols don't only protect plants. They can also protect you. Specifically, your brain. And as they benefit your brain, they relieve depression.

No one knows exactly how polyphenols work to ease and erase depression. But there are several theories, based on cellular and animal research. Here are some of the things polyphenols do:

- Regulate the levels of *norepinephrine* and *epinephrine*, neurotransmitters that direct the flow of information within the brain

- Limit the production of *glutamate*, an *excitatory* (stimulating) neurotransmitter that is toxic in large quantities

- Slow the production and release of *histamine*, a neurotransmitter and inflammatory biochemical released during allergic reactions

- Optimize levels of brain-derived neurotrophic factor (BDNF), a protein crucial for maintaining the health of neurons

- Protect the fat-rich cells of the brain from *lipid peroxidation*, a kind of internal rust generated by renegade molecules called *reactive oxygen species* or *free radicals*. These molecules are formed by pollutants, diets high in fat and sugar, stress, smoking, and other factors. Antioxidants like OPCs stabilize free radicals so that they do less damage.

- Strengthen and repair the delicate *blood-brain barrier*, keeping neurotoxins like pesticides and food additives out of the brain

- Improve blood flow to the brain, helping deliver crucial brain-supporting nutrients

- Balance brain waves. Imbalanced alpha waves (associated with relaxation and calm) are linked to depression.

- Absorb and disarm metals that can harm the brain, like lead

- Boost enzymes that decrease inflammation in the brain

There's plenty of real-world scientific proof to back up those theories. **Lower polyphenol intake, higher risk of depression.** Australian researchers analyzed results from thirty-seven studies on the role of polyphenols in the symptoms of depression, publishing their results in the May 1, 2020, issue of *Advances in Nutrition*. They reached two conclusions: 1) The lower your intake of polyphenols, the more likely you are to develop depression; and 2) adding polyphenols to the diet can effectively alleviate depressive symptoms.[1]

Twenty-seven percent lower risk of depressive symptoms. In a similar study, published in *Clinical Nutrition* in December 2022, French researchers studied more than one thousand people for fifteen years, and found that those with the highest intake of polyphenols had a 27 percent lower risk of depressive symptoms.[2]

Let's take a closer look at the most powerful OPCs and how they work to turn the tables on depression—and the best way to add these OPCs to your daily regimen, which is to combine many of them in *one* daily supplement.

Grape and Grape Seed Extracts: Feeling Fine on the Vine

Maybe you've heard of *resveratrol,* the OPC in grapes that is a powerful antioxidant and that has been touted for its ability to protect against heart disease, stroke, cancer, liver diseases, obesity, diabetes, Alzheimer's disease, and Parkinson's disease. Research on resveratrol shows it can also shield you from depression.

A bonus of well-being. In a twelve-month study involving 125 healthy postmenopausal women, researchers from Australia found that adding a resveratrol supplement to the diet led to decreased pain and improved "general well-being," including fewer depressive symptoms and better mood.[3]

Depressive symptoms—made much better. In summing up the research on resveratrol and depression, a team of scientists from America and Brazil concluded resveratrol may be "a potential anti-depressant agent" and may help "ameliorate depressive symptoms in humans."[4]

Resveratrol may be the most famous of grape polyphenols, but grapes contain many others. And they work to beat depression, too.

Red grape extract to the rescue. Italian researchers studied 111 healthy older adults, dividing them into two groups: one group took a supplement with grape polyphenols; the other took a placebo.[5]

At the start of the study, the participants took several tests to measure mental and emotional status: a test for detecting cognitive clarity and possible cognitive impairment; for depression; for anxiety; and for "neuropsychological status," which measures attention (focus), memory, and language skills. After twelve weeks, the researchers repeated the tests—and found supplementation was a success.

Compared to the placebo, the grape polyphenol supplement:

- decreased depression by 16 percent;

- decreased anxiety by 25 percent;

- improved cognitive clarity;

- improved concentration, and short- and long-term memory; and

- improved language skills, like verbal fluency.

A tonic for menopausal depression—and much more. In a study in *Menopause*, Japanese researchers tested ninety-one women aged forty to sixty who had at least one menopausal symptom, giving one group of women grape seed extract and another group a placebo. After two months, the women taking the grape seed extract had less depression and anxiety—as well as fewer hot flashes, less insomnia, lower blood pressure, and more muscle mass. Grape seed polyphenols are "effective in improving the physical and psychological symptoms of menopause," concluded the researchers.[6]

Don't rely on red wine. One important point about red grapes: Red wine is *not* a remedy for depression! For one thing, it can't deliver the level of polyphenols that make the difference. For another, wine itself (like all alcoholic drinks) *is* a depressant. Drinking red wine every day is not a sensible strategy for beating depression and improving mood.

Blueberries and Blueberry Extract: Fruitful Remedy

If you've got the blues, *eat* the blues—in the form of OPC-rich blueberries. Here's some of the science supporting that statement:

Thirty-three percent less depression. Researchers from England studied forty-five adults, dividing them into three groups. One group drank tart cherry juice; one group drank blueberry juice; and the third group received a placebo drink. After twenty days, those drinking the blueberry juice had a 33 percent decrease in depressive symptoms. They also had lower total and low-density lipoprotein (LDL) cholesterol.[7]

Preventing postpartum blues: Forty-four times less sadness—with blueberries. Canadian researchers studied forty-one pregnant women, giving twenty-one of them a dietary supplement that contained blueberry juice and blueberry extract (along with two neurotransmitter-

Finally Hopeful Success Story

PATIENT: Agnes

TREATED FOR: ADHD and depression

The OPCs that I discuss in this chapter are a foundational nutritional supplement for adults with ADHD, helping to balance brain waves.

One of the adults who benefited from OPCs was Agnes, a woman in her thirties with ADHD. She wasn't a patient of mine, but her nephew was. I was treating him for ADHD and had prescribed OPCs, which made a big difference. And seeing her nephew feel and act a lot better, she decided to try the supplement for herself.

Later, she wrote me to tell me what happened.

"I have had ADHD my whole life, but my depression started in my twenties, after a bad breakup. I was prescribed an antidepressant, but the side effects—weight gain, insomnia, low libido—weren't bearable. My depression eased somewhat but roared back in my thirties, and I refused to go back on antidepressants.

"Well, I was delighted when I took OPCs for my ADHD—and my mood brightened dramatically. After just a week or two, I felt like a huge weight had been lifted off my life.

"Thanks, Dr. Greenblatt!"

enhancing amino acids). On the fifth day after giving birth—the typical peak of postpartum blues—all forty-one women underwent a "sad mood induction procedure," a technique to trigger sad or negative emotions, using sad music, sad stories, and the like. In the women who didn't take blueberry, sad mood shot up by an average measure of 44 points—compared to virtually *no* increase in sadness (.05 points) in the blueberry group.

"This dietary supplement," wrote the researchers in the prestigious *Proceedings of the National Academies of Sciences*, "eliminates vulnerability to depressed mood during the peak of postpartum blues."[8]

Better memory—and mood. Researchers in the Department of Psychiatry at the University of Cincinnati studied nine older adults with memory loss. They had them drink a glass of blueberry juice every day for twelve weeks—and saw recall and learning improve. They also saw "reduced depressive symptoms."[9]

Boosts mood in kids, too. Researchers in England studied twenty-one kids aged eighteen to twenty-one, and fifty kids aged seven to ten. The kids got either a blueberry drink or a placebo. Right before imbibing the drink and two hours later, the researchers measured positive and negative emotions—and the kids getting the blueberry drink had a significant *increase* in positive emotions.[10]

Green Tea and Green Tea Extract: A Cup of Contentment

Green tea is rich in polyphenols. The most well studied is epigallocatechin gallate (EGCG), with research showing it is anti-inflammatory, anticancer, antidiabetic, anti-obesity, and good for the heart and immune system.

It's antidepressive, too—according to dozens of studies on thousands of people.

Let's look at two categories of those studies: *epidemiological* research, which analyzes health data from thousands of people; and *clinical* research, which uses green tea or a green tea extract as a treatment over a period of weeks or months. First, a small sampling of many epidemiological studies:

Sixty-six percent less risk of depressive symptoms. Japanese researchers analyzed the results of eight studies on green tea and depression—and found people with "high green tea consumption" lowered the risk of developing depressive symptoms by 66 percent. The results were reported in the *Journal of Nutritional Science and Vitaminology*.[11]

And in a four-year study of more than three thousand people, published in the *Journal of Nutrition, Health and Aging* in 2021, people who drank three or more cups of tea daily were 46 percent less likely to develop depression.[12]

One cup of tea, 61 percent less stress. In a study reported in the journal *Antioxidants* in January 2023, an international team of researchers analyzed health data from 1,572 adults. Those who drank one cup of tea (or coffee) daily were 61 percent less likely to feel under stress, and 56 percent less likely to have depressive symptoms. (Coffee is rich in chlorogenic acid, a powerful polyphenol that is also found in apples, pears, eggplant, and tomatoes.)[13]

Now on to the clinical research:

Fewer depressive symptoms—with green tea extract. Fifty people with mild to moderate depression took either green tea extract or a placebo for twelve weeks—and those who took the extract had significantly fewer depressive symptoms. Green tea extract could be a therapy for mild to moderate depression, concluded the researchers, in *Chinese Herbal Medicine*.[14]

L-theanine—unique relief in green tea. Green tea contains uniquely high levels of L-theanine, a calming and relaxing amino acid. Patients taking L-theanine were shown to have increased alpha waves, the brain waves linked to a state of restful alertness. (Practitioners of Zen bred green tea to contain high levels of L-theanine in order to improve their meditation.)

In a study from Japanese researchers, twenty people with major depressive disorder (MDD) had 250 milligrams (mg) per day of L-theanine added to their treatment regimen of antidepressant medication. After eight weeks, the patients had fewer depressive symptoms and less anxiety than those who didn't take L-theanine. They also had improved cognitive function, including better memory. And they slept better, too.[15]

And in a study published in the July 2023 issue of the *Journal of Affective Disorders*, fifty people with MDD received either Zoloft and L-theanine or Zoloft and a placebo. After six weeks, those receiving both Zoloft *and* L-theanine had "remarkable symptom improvement."[16]

Fourteen days to better moods. Japanese researchers studied the effect of green tea on "depression-like moods" in eighty-one people, reporting their results in the journal *Nutrients* in 2022. They found a "significant improvement in depressive tendencies" after people drank green tea regularly for two weeks. The participants also had much less anxiety.

Green tea, they conclude, "can improve depressed mood"—and they theorize it works by decreasing inflammation and easing the body's response to stress.[17]

How green tea works to relieve depression. A review of "the antidepressant potential" of tea in the August 2022 issue of *Food Research International* also speculates about mechanism of action, with Chinese researchers suggesting several probable ways that tea fights depression.[18] Green tea:

1. calms the hypothalamic-pituitary-adrenal (HPA) axis, which regulates the body's response to stress;

2. reduces inflammation;

3. restores the system that generates the neurotransmitters serotonin, dopamine, and norepinephrine;

4. lowers levels of monoamine oxidase, which breaks down those three neurotransmitters; and

5. improves communication between the gut microbiome and the brain.

Pine Bark:
Recovering Your Stolen Libido

Pine bark extract is loaded with OPCs—and research shows it can help osteoarthritis, diabetes, high blood pressure, perimenopausal symptoms, ADHD, heart disease, asthma, and cognitive function.

It can also help men and women recover a libido that's been stolen by antidepressant medication.

Yes, so-called "sexual dysfunction" is a common side effect of antidepressants—with a paper in the *Journal of Clinical Psychiatry*[19] showing that six out of ten people taking an antidepressant develop this problem. And 60 percent is a conservative figure. In one study cited in the paper, 93 percent of men and women taking Anafranil (clomipramine) suffered from either partial or total anorgasmia, the inability to have an orgasm.[20]

The types of sexual side effects caused by antidepressants include: less sexual desire (low libido); less sexual excitement (and even complete loss of sensation in the penis or vagina); diminished or delayed orgasm; erectile dysfunction; and painful ejaculation. Talk about depressing!

Pine bark extract might help you get your groove back.

After one month—fewer sexual side effects. In a study published in the March 1, 2019, issue of *Physiology International*, researchers in eastern Europe studied seventy-two people with depression who were taking Lexapro. They divided them into two groups: Thirty-seven took Lexapro *and* Pycnogenol, a pine bark extract; thirty-five continued to take Lexapro only.[21]

After one month of treatment, those who were taking Pycnogenol had much less sexual dysfunction.

The researchers speculate the pine bark extract worked by improving circulation and reducing inflammation.

And pine bark extract may help not only with low libido—it may help improve mood itself.

In an eight-week study of thirty-eight women with menopausal symptoms, Pycnogenol effectively treated loss of libido—and mood swings, hot flashes, night sweats, and vaginal dryness.[22]

Rhodiola Rosea

Soothing the Stress That Triggers Depression

Rhodiola rosea is a hardy herb from the arctic regions of Siberia, Scandinavia, and Canada. It normalizes the body's response to stress and is an effective tonic for relieving mental and physical fatigue. It's good for enhancing concentration, and I often use it in the treatment of ADHD. And it stops the breakdown of the neurotransmitters dopamine and norepinephrine, improving depressive symptoms.

In a study in the *Nordic Journal of Psychiatry*, eighty-nine people with mild to moderate depression were divided into three groups. Group One took 680 mg of *Rhodiola* daily; Group Two took 1,360 mg daily; and Group Three took a placebo. After six weeks, those taking the *Rhodiola* "improved significantly" in "overall depression" and "emotional instability."[23]

For depression, I typically start a patient on 100 mg per day of *Rhodiola rosea*, slowly increasing up to a maximum of 400 mg daily, adding 100 mg per week. (In other words: Week 1, 100 mg; Week 2, 200 mg; Week 3, 300 mg; Week 4, 400 mg.) Some individuals notice improvement at 100 mg, while others may need more.

Rhodiola rosea is safe, but there are a few precautions. If you have been diagnosed with bipolar disorder, *Rhodiola* isn't for you: it might make mania worse.

As for buying *Rhodiola rosea*: Buyer beware! Testing shows that many herbal products don't contain the amount of herb promised on the label. It's always best to do some personal research and find a reputable supplement company, perhaps subscribing to a service like consumerlab.com, which publishes reviews of nutritional and herbal supplements, or checking customer reviews in a supplement category you're investigating.

Curcumin:
Gold-Standard Depression Relief

Curcumin is the active ingredient in turmeric, the popular, gold-colored spice in the cuisine of India. It's uniquely rich in anti-inflammatory and antioxidant polyphenols, and it's been shown to protect and improve the health of virtually every organ of the body—including the brain.

In fact, thousands of animal and human studies from around the world have found that curcumin can combat more than seventy disorders and diseases, like cancer, heart disease, type 2 diabetes, Alzheimer's disease—and depression. (And when it comes to turmeric, modern science is just getting on the bandwagon. Use of turmeric compounds in Ayurveda, the ancient natural healing system of India, dates back nearly four thousand years.)

How does curcumin work to protect and heal your brain? In many ways:

As an antioxidant, it protects neurons from the cell-damaging free radicals produced by oxidation; protects mitochondria, the tiny energy factories in every cell; and guards against DNA damage. It also boosts antioxidant enzymes, like superoxide dismutase.

As an anti-inflammatory, it decreases a host of pro-inflammatory compounds like COX-2 and TNF-alpha; balances the kynurenine pathway in the brain, which helps decrease neuroinflammation; increases the sensitivity of the peroxisome proliferator–activated receptor (PPAR), yet another way of cooling inflammation; and regulates microglia, immune cells in the brain.

As a neuroprotective compound, it increases BDNF, nerve growth factor (NGF), and glial cell line-derived neurotrophic factor (GDNF), three "growth factors" that keep neurons healthy; helps preserve neuronal stem cells, which help repair or replace damaged neurons; improves the "complexity" of synapses—the junctions between neurons—aiding in signaling within the brain; increases levels of acetylcholinesterase, an enzyme that regulates neurotransmission; and helps synthesize neurotrophin, proteins that helps neurons develop, survive, and grow.

Scientific studies show that all of these mechanisms of action work together to produce powerful antidepressive effects. The results from a few of those studies:

In diabetes, less depression and anxiety. People with diabetes have triple the risk of depression compared to nondiabetics. In a clinical study, eighty patients with diabetes were divided into two groups, with half taking curcumin and half taking a placebo. After eight weeks, those taking curcumin had an 8 percent drop in depression and anxiety scores.[24]

Curcumin supplementation "was effective in reducing depression and anxiety," concluded the researchers, in *Phytotherapy Research.*

Significant antidepressant effects. In a twelve-week study from Thailand, sixty-five people with major depression received either curcumin (500 to 1,500 mg per day) or a placebo. Curcumin "has significant antidepressant effects," concluded the researchers in *Neurotoxicity Research.*[25]

Improvements in depressive symptoms. Researchers in Australia studied 123 people with major depressive disorder, giving them either low-dose curcumin (250 mg per day), high-dose curcumin (500 mg per day), or a placebo. Those taking the curcumin had "significantly greater improvements in depressive symptoms" than those taking the placebo, wrote the researchers in the *Journal of Affective Disorders.* The treatment was particularly effective in people with atypical depression, which includes symptoms like overeating and insomnia.[26]

Boosting the power of antidepressants. One hundred eight depressed men had curcumin or a placebo added to their treatment regimen. "Supplementation with curcumin produced significant antidepressant behavior response," wrote the researchers in the *Journal of Clinical Psychopharmacology.*[27]

Ten studies rate curcumin a "10" for depression. A 2020 study by Italian psychiatrists analyzed the results from ten other studies on curcumin and depression, involving 531 people—and found that curcumin added to standard care "might improve depressive symptoms in people with depression."[28]

And an earlier meta-analysis, from 2017, reporting on six studies with 377 patients, found "significant clinical efficacy of curcumin in ameliorating depressive symptoms."[29]

Treatment with OPCs

Over the decades, I've slowly but surely found the best way to treat with OPCs: Use a *combination* of OPCs rather than just one. The combined OPC supplement I use in my practice is one I formulated myself: CurcumaSorb Mind, from Pure Encapsulations. It contains many of the OPCs we've discussed here: grape extract, blueberry extract, green tea extract, and pine bark extract. It also contains curcumin.

You might notice that the form of pine bark extract in this supplement is not Pycnogenol, which is from French maritime pine; it's an extract from Monterey pine. In my experience, Monterey pine bark extract works just as well as Pycnogenol but is far less expensive.

I recommend two multi-OPC pills a day, one with breakfast, one with dinner.

As for safety: in twenty-five years of treating patients with OPCs, I've rarely seen a negative side effect.

If you decide to take curcumin separately, I recommend the well-studied (and well-absorbed) formulations Theracurmin or Meriva. (Research shows that Theracurmin is up to twenty-seven times more bioavailable than other curcumin supplements, and Meriva is up to twenty-nine times more bioavailable.) Take Theracurmin at 60 to 180 mg per day, or Meriva at 500 to 2,000 mg per day.

For maximum absorbability, take your curcumin supplement with or shortly after a meal or a snack.

STEP-BY-STEP ACTION PLAN FOR

Polyphenols

Use this practical, step-by-step summary to implement the therapeutic actions discussed in this chapter.

OPCs

Step #1: Take a supplement with a combination of OPCs. I recommend the product I formulated: CurcumaSorb Mind, from Pure Encapsulations. It contains grape extract, blueberry extract, green tea extract, pine bark extract, and curcumin.

Dosage: Take two pills daily, one with breakfast, one with dinner.

Curcumin

Step #1: If you take curcumin separately, I recommend the brands Theracurmin or Meriva, both of which are well absorbed.

Dosage: Theracurmin, 60 to 180 mg per day. Meriva, 500 to 2,000 mg per day. For maximum absorbability, take with a meal or snack.

Rhodiola

Step #1: Start with 100 mg per day, slowly increasing up to a maximum of 400 mg daily, adding 100 mg per week.

Precaution: Don't take *Rhodiola* if you have been diagnosed with bipolar disorder. It might make mania worse.

PART THREE

MEDICAL CARE, BEHAVIORAL CARE, AND SELF-CARE

CHAPTER 11

Repairing the Gut-Brain Network

> Gut feelings are very real—in fact, your gut may be the master controller of your moods!

"All disease begins in the gut."

So said Hippocrates—the Greek "father of medicine"—2,500 years ago.

Two thousand five hundred years later, a growing number of doctors and medical researchers are agreeing with him—and finding that "all disease" includes depression. Moreover, they're finding that the link between the gut and the brain is very strong.

The Gut-Brain Axis

There is new scientific insight into an internal, two-way network called the "gut-brain axis"—a network by which the gut directly influences what happens in the brain (and vice versa). The components of this gut-brain axis include:

The gut microbiome. The gut is home to trillions of microorganisms collectively known as the *gut microbiome*. Among the more than five hundred species of bacteria, many are friendly—meaning, they're indispensable to health. These bacteria perform *many* crucial functions.

You can thank friendly bacteria for:

- digesting protein;

- digesting milk sugar (lactose);

- increasing the absorption of minerals;

- manufacturing vitamins B and K;

- manufacturing essential fatty acids (EFAs) and short-chain fatty acids (SCFAs); and

- preventing *dysbiosis*, the overgrowth of bad bacteria.

But you can also thank the friendly bacteria for positive mood—with studies now showing that supplements containing these friendly bacteria (probiotics) are so powerful they can *treat* depression. (More about probiotic treatment later in this chapter.)

How can the microbial composition of the gut influence the activity of the brain? Because the balance between friendly and unfriendly bacteria influences *all* of the other components of the gut-brain axis:

The enteric nervous system (ENS). Often referred to as the "second brain," this complex network of neurons is embedded in the lining of the gastrointestinal tract. It contains over one hundred million neurons—more than the spinal cord. And it can operate independently of the central nervous system (the brain and spinal cord), playing a direct role in regulating digestive processes—and mood.

Put another way: the nervous system in the gut is in direct communication with the central nervous system. If digestion is bad, it's likely you'll feel bad—depressed and anxious. It's likely that your thinking will be foggy, too, with poor concentration and weak memory.

Neurotransmitters. The ENS uses more than thirty neurotransmitters to communicate neuron to neuron—just like the brain. Serotonin, gamma-aminobutyric acid (GABA), norepinephrine, dopamine—all these mood-related neurotransmitters are found in the gut. And not just in tiny amounts. *Ninety-five percent* of the body's serotonin is found in the gut, with the remaining 5 percent in the brain. Changes in the gut affect neurotransmitter levels in the gut—which, in turn, directly affects the brain.

Hormones. Not only is there an extensive nervous system in the gut, there's also an extensive hormone-generating endocrine system—the enteric endocrine system. And these hormones send a host of mood-modulating signals along the gut-brain axis to the brain.

Immune system. Seventy percent of the cells of the immune system are in (you guessed it) the gut—in the mucosal immune system. And these immune cells—and the inflammatory signals they send out when you have dysbiosis—can influence the brain. In fact, many experts theorize that gut inflammation—and the brain inflammation it triggers—may be the primary way gut problems lead to depression.

Vagus nerve. This long nerve connects the brainstem to the abdomen and sends signals in both directions. Of note, 90 percent of the nerve fibers in the vagus nerve carry information *from* the gut and *to* the brain, not the other way round, demonstrating the importance of the gut in determining brain health.

The hypothalamic-pituitary-adrenal (HPA) axis. This neuroendocrine (nerve/hormone) system regulates your body's "fight-or-flight" response to stress, generating hormones (epinephrine/adrenaline, in particular) that clench muscles, speed heart rate, tighten arteries, muffle pain, pump out blood sugar—and shut down digestion. (You don't want to be digesting food when you're running away from a saber-toothed tiger.)

The fight-or-flight response is a necessary way of handling short-term stress. But *chronic stress* keeps the HPA activated, interfering with gut function. And the digestive problems caused by chronic stress can worsen depression.

As I said at the beginning of this section, the gut microbiome influences *all* of the above factors—the ENS, gut neurotransmitters, gut hormones, the immune system in the gut, the vagus nerve, and the HPA axis.

Which means if you have dysbiosis, your brain is going to hear about it!

Probiotic Therapy

I'm going into so much detail about the gut-brain axis to give you the best possible picture of just how important your gut is to your brain and your mood—and to motivate you to manage your gut health.

So, exactly how do you prevent or reverse dysbiosis, and give friendly bacteria the upper hand?

Well, you can consume more fermented, probiotic-rich foods, like yogurt, kefir, buttermilk, cottage cheese, sauerkraut, kimchi, sour pick-

---

Case in Point: Irritable Bowel Syndrome (IBS)

A good illustration of the gut-brain axis at work: IBS, which one scientific paper calls "a microbiome-gut-brain axis disorder."

The symptoms of IBS include constipation and/or diarrhea, gas, and abdominal bloating and cramping.

IBS is almost always accompanied by dysbiosis. Dysbiosis inflames the gut's immune system, and increases gut permeability (leaky gut syndrome), further inflaming the body. Dysbiosis also activates sensory pathways that increase gut pain. All of these factors affect the brain, which then interferes with the speed of digestion (causing the diarrhea or constipation), increases sensitivity to pain, and further alters the nervous, hormonal, and immune systems in the gut, in a vicious cycle.

While all that is happening in IBS, emotions are riled up, too. Depression affects 27 percent of people with IBS, and anxiety affects 38 percent—*double* the rate of depression and anxiety in people without IBS.

Or as one research paper put it, in the formal language of science: IBS often involves psychological comorbidities associated with the alteration of the gut microbiome.

Well, that's the case for *any* kind of digestive upset and disease.

les, miso soup, tempeh, raw honey, and kombucha, a fermented, effervescent tea. (But introduce fermented foods *gradually*, to avoid gas and bloating.) You can also eat foods rich in prebiotics, food ingredients that nourish the probiotics in the gut, like vegetables, fruit, and beans.

Consuming more probiotics and prebiotics is a good idea. But going on a probiotic-rich diet as therapy for depression is unlikely to make a significant difference if you are struggling with depression. And even if diet could make a difference, most people find it difficult to sustain a specific dietary regimen.

Taking probiotic *supplements* for depression is simpler and more reliable. And it's sustainable on a daily basis. Plus, it's what has worked in my clinical practice. And not just in my practice. The science of using probiotic supplements for mental health has advanced to the point where such probiotics are called *psychobiotics*—the use of specific strains of probiotics that affect mood, behavior, and cognition.

A recent scientific paper in the journal *Cureus*, from researchers at Wayne State University Detroit Medical Center, sums up the current state of knowledge about using probiotics to treat depression.[1] The researchers stated:

1. There is a significant relationship between the composition and alteration of the gut microbiome and the presence of symptoms of depression.

2. Treatment with probiotics or prebiotics improved the symptoms of depression.

3. Treatment with probiotics or prebiotics may decrease the severity of depression by altering the gut microbiome.

Let's look at a few individual studies featured in that article and elsewhere.

Depression reduced by 50 percent—with probiotics. In a study published in the April 2019 issue of *Clinical Nutrition*, researchers divided eighty-one people with major depressive disorder (MDD) who were taking antidepressants into three groups: one group received a probiotic supplement; one, a prebiotic supplement; and one, a placebo. After eight weeks, the probiotic group had a 50 percent decrease in depressive symptoms. The prebiotic and placebo groups had little change.[2]

Probiotics boost the power of Prozac. In a study published in the *Archives of Neuroscience* in 2018, researchers studied forty patients with moderate depression. The patients took Prozac for four weeks, and then took either a "synbiotic" or a placebo for the next six weeks. (Probiotic supplements can contain both probiotics and prebiotics, a combo that is called a synbiotic.) The synbiotic group had a "clinically significant decrease" in depression compared to the placebo group.[3]

Probiotics help depression in IBS—and reduce stress. In a study published in the August 2017 issue of *Gastroenterology*, an international team of researchers gave forty-four people with IBS either a probiotic or a placebo. After six weeks, 67 percent of the IBS patients taking a probiotic had a significant decrease in depression scores—compared to 35 percent of the placebo group. The patients taking the probiotic also had an improvement in quality of life compared to the placebo group. (In scientific studies, quality of life reflects several factors, like physical health, mental health, social relationships, and personal satisfaction.) The study produced another interesting finding:

The participants had their brains scanned while looking at images of fearful faces—and those taking the probiotic had reduced activity in their amygdala, the part of the brain that processes fear. In other words, the probiotic group was less stressed out when they looked at stressful images.[4]

Probiotics help postpartum depression (PPD). In research published in the October 2017 issue of *EbioMedicine*, scientists from New Zealand studied 380 pregnant women, giving them either a probiotic or a placebo from fifteen weeks into their pregnancy until six months after they gave birth. Women in the probiotic group had 22 percent lower depression scores than the placebo group. They also had less anxiety.[5]

A meta-analysis of eighteen papers on depression and probiotics shows—probiotics work. In a study published in the August 2023 issue of *Nutrients*, Spanish researchers analyzed results from eighteen studies on depression and probiotics. Their conclusion: "A combination of different probiotic strains . . . could be a good mixture as an adjuvant [addition] in the treatment of depressive disorders."[6]

That's my conclusion, too.

The Probiotic Protocol

Testing for dysbiosis might be a good idea if you have depression and gastrointestinal woes. I use the Organic Acid Test (OAT) urine test, which detects bacteria and fungal imbalances in the gut.

But even without testing, I think *everybody* who is depressed can benefit from taking a daily probiotic. The benefits go way beyond your gut and brain, with studies showing probiotic supplementation can help treat heart disease, type 2 diabetes, obesity, fatty liver disease, polycystic ovary syndrome (PCOS), gout, a range of gut problems, and even improve the efficacy of radiation treatment in cancer.

Look for a probiotic supplement that delivers twenty to fifty billion colony-forming units (CFU). Take the supplement two times daily, with or without food, per the supplement manufacturer's recommendation.

There are two products I routinely recommend to my patients:

- Probiotic G.I. from Pure Encapsulations, which delivers a combination of *Lactobacillus acidophilus, Lactobacillus salivarius, Lactobacillus casei, Bifidobacterium bifidum, Bifidobacterium lactis*, and *Streptococcus thermophilus*.

- Ther-Biotic Metabolic Formula, from SFI Health.

Celiac Disease and Depression

Celiac disease (CD) is an *autoimmune disease*, in which the body's immune system attacks *gluten*—a protein found in wheat, rye, barley, and some types of oats—as a foreign invader. This attack causes inflammation—and damage to the digestive tract. Specifically, celiac disease damages and shrinks the *villi*, small, fingerlike projections that line the inner surface of the small intestine, providing a vast surface area for the absorption of nutrients.

Celiac disease affects one in 133 Americans.

Typically, the disease doesn't start at birth. It often doesn't appear until adulthood, when it's triggered by stress, gastrointestinal surgery, a viral infection, pregnancy, or other body-disturbing factors.

The classic symptoms of celiac include diarrhea, constipation, abdominal pain, intestinal gas, bloating, fatigue, and weight loss, along with non-gastrointestinal symptoms like joint pain, bone loss, skin rashes, oral ulcers—and depression.

The tragedy of celiac disease is that 83 percent of people with the problem are either undiagnosed, or misdiagnosed with other conditions. That's not so surprising when you also know that 50 percent or more of celiac patients have *few* or *no* symptoms. But they may have multiple nutritional deficiencies, leading to depression. In fact, poor absorption of nutrients—amino acids, vitamins, minerals, and EFAs—is a *major* consequence of celiac disease.

In one study of celiac patients on a long-term, gluten-free diet, researchers found deficiencies in:[7]

- vitamin B12 (30 percent);

- iron (40 percent);

- folate (20 percent);

- vitamin D (25 percent); and

- zinc (40 percent).

These deficiencies are caused not only by poor absorption, but by lowered nutritional intake from a gluten-free diet and eating more processed foods.

This link between celiac disease and nutritional deficiency is so marked that the American College of Gastroenterology recommends that physicians test *all* newly diagnosed CD patients for nutritional deficiencies—and supplement as necessary to correct the deficiencies.

Eating a Gluten-Free Diet

If you have celiac disease, removing gluten from your diet is the *only* way to stop ongoing damage to your intestines and give your body the chance to heal.

That means you stop eating all foods containing gluten, including wheat, rye, oats, and barley, and anything made from them. The task can be complex because gluten is used as a thickening and stabilizing agent, showing up in many foods. Obvious ones include:

- baking mixes;
- beer;
- bread;
- cakes and pies;
- pretzels;
- cereal;
- cookies/crackers;
- pastries;
- doughnuts;
- muffins; and
- pasta.

But a number of nonobvious foods can also contain gluten, including:

- ice cream;
- ketchup;
- soy sauce;
- licorice;
- sauces (thickened with flour);
- salad dressings;
- chutneys and pickles;
- instant cocoa;
- processed meats;
- meat substitutes; and
- spices (with anticaking agents).

If the diet seems challenging, consider working with a dietician experienced in helping people create and stay on a gluten-free eating style.

The proven link

Research shows that celiac disease and mental illness are often found together.

A 2021 study from the *Indian Journal of Gastroenterology* analyzed thirteen studies on CD and mental illness, and found CD increased the risk for major depression, persistent depressive disorder (PDD), anxiety, and panic disorder.[8]

In a study in the *Journal of Pediatric Gastroenterology and Nutrition*, 39 percent of 175 children and adolescents with biopsy-proven CD had significant concerns about their depression and/or anxiety.[9]

In a study published in *Cureus* in 2023, 83 percent of adults with CD had depression, and 85 percent had anxiety.[10]

Non-celiac gluten sensitivity

The link between gluten and depression goes beyond celiac disease.

An estimated two to three times more people—possibly as many as one in eight Americans—are sensitive to gluten but do *not* meet the diagnostic criteria for celiac.

And those folks not only have gastrointestinal symptoms like abdominal pain and bloating; they also have brain-based symptoms, like depression and brain fog.

Bottom line: If you have bowel issues and you're depressed—you should be tested for celiac disease. Even if celiac is *not* detected, you should consider a period of gluten-free eating, to see if your gut issues *and* depression are eased.

Your doctor can use a blood test to detect antibodies to gluten—if they're found, you may have an indication of the disease. But the definitive test for CD is a biopsy of the small intestine.

If celiac disease is confirmed, you should:

1. Eat a gluten-free diet.

2. Take probiotics, because everyone with celiac disease has dysbiosis.

3. Have comprehensive testing for nutritional deficiencies, which are common in celiac disease (and could be contributing to depression), and correct the deficiencies with targeted nutritional supplementation.

Clearing up *Candida*

Often, an obvious problem with your *physical health* provides the clue that allows you to discover the underlying cause of a *mental health* problem, like depression. For example:

Do you have recurrent fungal infections? I'm talking about problems like:

Thickened, discolored, crumbly, fungus-infected toenails. Athlete's foot. Fungal infections in the groin area, buttocks, or inner thighs, commonly called jock itch. Yeast infection of the vagina. (*Yeast* is a type of fungi.) Fungal infections in skin folds, like under the breasts.

All these recurrent, persistent *outer* infections could be a sign of an *inner* infection—an overgrowth in your gut of the fungus *Candida albicans*. (The medical name for the condition is *candidiasis*.) And that overgrowth could be bad news for your mood and motivation. Because when *Candida* runs rampant in the gut, it can produce several neurotoxins, like acetaldehyde and ethanol. Those internal poisons can leak out of the gut and into the bloodstream, entering the brain, where they can spark neuroinflammation, disrupt neurotransmitters—and trigger or worsen depressive symptoms, including low mood, poor sleep, physical and mental fatigue, difficulty concentrating, and irritability.

Research supports the connection.

In one study, scientists looked at women with recurrent yeast infections and found they were "significantly more likely to suffer clinical depression."

In a 2024 study published in *Translational Psychiatry*, researchers analyzed health data from more than five hundred thousand people and found that people with major depression were 52 percent more likely to have a *Candida* infection.[11]

A study of more than eleven thousand women in the *Journal of Psy-*

Finally Hopeful Success Story

PATIENT: Stanley

TREATMENT FOR: Depression—and Celiac Disease

Stanley was a forty-four-year-old lawyer on disability due to chronic depression. After trying more than a dozen different medications, and multiple rounds of transcranial magnetic stimulation, Stanley was still struggling with overwhelming symptoms. When I saw him in my office, his depression had crippled his ability to work. His day was filled with visits to therapists, counselors, and physicians. His once-promising career had been derailed by severe depression.

My initial laboratory testing showed that Stanley had low levels of vitamins D, B12 and iron, and was borderline anemic. Naturally, I was curious about his diet. Stanley said he had been following a paleo diet, focusing on red meat, chicken, and non-starchy vegetables. Because he ate a lot of meat and still had low iron levels, I suspected malabsorption—and ordered a test for celiac disease.

Stanley tested positive. My diagnosis: Major depression, secondary to celiac disease.

chiatric Research showed a similar link, with the authors finding that candidiasis had a "significant association with depression."[12]

If I see a patient with persistent fungal infections, I order the Organic Acid Test (the OAT) to see if they have breakdown products of *Candida* in their gut.

But there are many times when I don't order this test—I simply treat a depressed person with recurrent fungal infections as if they have *Candida* overgrowth in the gut. In this case, the Functional Psychiatry Treatment Plan typically consists of:

1. **Probiotics.** I often put a depressed patient with suspected *Candida* overgrowth on the probiotic *Saccharomyces boulardii* (five

Stanley's Functional Psychiatry Treatment Plan consisted of:

- vitamin D, 5,000 international units (IU) daily;
- B12 injections, 1,000 mcg weekly;
- iron bisglycinate, 20 mg, three times daily;
- Zinc, 30 mg;
- a multivitamin; and
- a gluten-free diet.

With the implementation of the Plan, and a gluten-free diet, Stanley's recovery was slow but steady. After three months, his depression symptoms were improved enough that he was able to return to work. Testing also showed his nutritional deficiencies were resolved. We stopped the B12 injections, iron, and zinc, but continued with vitamin D and the multivitamin.

As I discuss in this chapter, celiac disease is an often-overlooked cause or contributing factor to depression (and other mental health problems). If you and your doctor find that testing reveals significant nutritional deficiencies—test for celiac disease.

billion CFU, four times a day)—which, strangely enough, is itself a yeast. But just as there are good and bad bacteria, there are good and bad yeasts—and *S. boulardii* is a good yeast that can crowd out the bad, regulating gut health and protecting the gut from toxins.

2. **More antifungal food and spices.** Antifungal foods include coconut, garlic, oregano, and ginger. They are definitely *not* lightweights when it comes to battling *Candida*—several laboratory studies show that garlic extract, gingerroot, and oregano oil are just as powerful at killing *Candida* as Nystatin, an antifungal medication.

3. **Less sugar.** The sweet stuff is *Candida's* favorite food and fuels its growth. The less refined sugar in your diet, the better.

Infections Can Bring You Down

You know how you feel when you have an *acute infection*, like a cold or flu. You're fatigued and lethargic, with little or no motivation. Your appetite is poor, and your sleep is disturbed. And you probably feel down in the dumps, with a blah mood.

In other words, the symptoms of an acute infection mimic some of the symptoms of depression.

That's not a coincidence. There is a *biochemical* reason why infection and depression go hand in hand.

When you have a cold or flu, the body's immune system produces *cytokines*, proteins that help fight infection. Those cytokines also affect the brain, triggering negative changes in mood. And the main way cytokines compromise the brain is by triggering *neuroinflammation*.

Inflammation is an integral part of the healing process. It helps stop the spread of pathogens like bacteria and viruses, increases needed blood flow to the infected area, cleans up debris generated by infection, and regenerates tissue. And once healing is complete—like the ten to fourteen days of a cold or flu—inflammation (including neuroinflammation) is supposed to fade away.

But when you have a *chronic infection*, inflammation (including neuroinflammation) doesn't exit the scene. It simmers, producing a continuous, elevated output of inflammatory cytokines that can damage tissue, including the brain—causing or complicating depression.

Unfortunately, chronic infections are almost always overlooked as possible causes of depression. And that's a big problem. Because some people with depression make a *dramatic recovery* when an underlying chronic infection is found and fixed.

4. **Caprylic acid.** This coconut oil extract is a powerful antifungal, and a clinically proven treatment for *Candida* overgrowth. For more effectiveness, combine it with thymol and carvacrol (components of oregano oil). A study in *Cellular Physiology & Biochemistry* found this combination doubled caprylic acid's *Candida*-defeating power.[13] A product containing all three components is Candida Support, by NOW Foods.

5. **Nystatin.** This prescription oral antifungal medication works locally in the gut, and is not absorbed into the body, making it a reasonable choice for treating *Candida* overgrowth. Talk to your primary care physician about this medication.

Bottom line: If you're depressed *and* have a persistent fungal infection, talk to your doctor about this protocol.

Bottom line: As you partner with a physician to help you overcome depression, consider the possibility that a chronic infection—like *Candida*, Lyme disease, or Long COVID—might be contributing to or causing your depressive symptoms.

How to Nourish Your Friendly Bacteria and Your Brain: Don't Eat Ultra-Processed Foods (UPFs)

I recently saw an ebook from a fellow psychiatrist that offered a nutritional program to beat depression—a program based mostly on diet. I understand the intention was positive, but here's the truth:

Depression is a biological, brain-based problem that often reflects nutritional deficiencies. And these deficiencies are not always correctable by diet alone.

To overcome these depression-causing deficiencies, you need:

1) Testing, to *find* the deficiency.

2) Supplementation, to *fix* the deficiency.

Find and fix is the functional approach of this book—a proven approach that has worked over many decades, for thousands of patients.

Throughout Part I, I discuss *why* depression-causing nutritional deficiencies are not correctable by diet. For one thing, very few people are able to consistently eat a nutrient-rich diet. Then there are the genetic factors that block the utilization of key nutrients, like folate. Aging dramatically cuts the absorption of many nutrients, like vitamin B12. Chronic stress burns up a nutrient faster than you can replace it with diet, like magnesium. That's not to mention nutrient-robbing chronic disease, environmental toxins, depleted soil, and sugary food. These and many other factors make diet *very* problematic as a cure for a chronic condition.

However, even though diet isn't usually sufficient to treat depression on its own, it can help you optimize brain health and mental well-being.

A dietary pattern that emphasizes *whole, minimally processed foods*— like the Mediterranean diet pattern or the DASH diet pattern—is the best way to nourish your brain.

But the healthiest dietary pattern may reflect not so much what you eat but what you don't eat: Ultra-processed foods (UPFs).

What are UPFs? An ultra-processed food has been, well, *processed*— stripped of most or all of its natural nutrients and fiber, with lots of sugar, fat, salt, and artificial ingredients added.

It's not that these added ingredients aren't tasty. In fact, they're so tasty that they affect the brain like cocaine or heroin, literally addicting you to the food—whether it's fast food, salty chips, doughnuts, a frozen meal, or some other packaged, convenient food.

These addictive, high-calorie, high-fat, high-sugar, high-salt, low-nutrient foods taste really *good*. But they're really bad for you *if* they make up the majority of your diet. And that's the case for many Americans.

UPFs make up about 60 percent of the calories in the average American diet—contributing to the chronic conditions and diseases that afflict so many of us, like obesity, high blood pressure, heart disease, stroke, type 2 diabetes, cancer, and Alzheimer's disease. (Not to mention digestive ills, chronic pain like arthritis, immune weakness, and on and on.)

And UPFs are also bad for your brain.

In a 2022 study of more than ten thousand American adults, the more UPFs they ate, the more likely they were to report mild depression or anxiety—confirming a decade of research into this connection.[14]

Another recent study, from Brazilian researchers, links UPFs to cognitive decline—a 28 percent faster rate of decline in people who consume more than 20 percent of their calories from UPFs.[15]

But here's the kicker in that study: the researchers found that if you followed a pattern of healthy eating like the Mediterranean diet—rich in whole grains, green leafy vegetables, legumes, nuts, berries, fish, chicken, and olive oil—you greatly reduced the risk from dementia *even if* your diet included some UPFs.

Plus, ultra-processed foods make it ultra-likely you'll suffer from dysbiosis, according to a study published in *Food Research International* in May 2023.[16]

Bottom line: Maximize whole foods, minimize UPFs.

How do you know if a food is a UPF?

Read the label. If there is a long list of ingredients—especially unpronounceable chemicals you would never use in home cooking—the food is likely to be a UPF. Likewise, if it's loaded with added sugar, fat, and/or salt, and low in essential nutrients—it's likely to be a UPF.

Another handy way of identifying UPFs is by using the "NOVA" scale, which was developed by researchers to define processing for nutritional studies. It consists of four tiers:

Tier 1: Unprocessed or minimally processed food, including natural, whole foods that have undergone minimal or no processing, like fruits, vegetables, legumes, nuts, seeds, eggs, milk, and fresh or frozen meat and fish. Make most of your food choices from *this* tier.

Tier 2: Processed culinary ingredients derived from unprocessed foods or nature, such as oils, butter, sugar, salt, and vinegar. Go for it! These are the ingredients that enhance flavor and improve texture.

Tier 3: Processed foods, which have undergone some processing and contain added ingredients, like canned fruits and vegetables, freshly made bread, cheese, and simple processed meats like cured ham or bacon. These foods are also on the menu.

Tier 4: UPFs, which includes highly processed foods that are typically manufactured using numerous additives, and which are usually ready-to-eat or require minimal preparation, and are high in unhealthy fats, sugars, salt, and artificial additives. Minimize these foods!

Hang out on Tiers 1, 2, and 3—and only spend a little time on Tier 4.

Repairing the Gut-Brain Network

Use this practical, step-by-step summary to implement the therapeutic actions discussed in this chapter.

Dysbiosis (imbalance of gut bacteria)

Step #1: Take a daily probiotic supplement, whether you have dysbiosis or not. Look for a supplement that delivers twenty to fifty billion CFUs. Take the supplement twice daily, with or without food.

Step #2: Eat more fermented probiotic-rich foods, like yogurt, sauerkraut, and sour pickles. Also eat foods rich in prebiotics (nutrients that nourish the probiotics in your gut), like vegetables, fruits, and beans.

Step #3: Eat fewer ultra-processed foods, like fast food, salty chips, doughnuts, and other types of packaged convenient foods. Maximize whole foods, like fruits, vegetables, legumes, nuts, seeds, eggs, milk, and fresh or frozen meat and fish.

CD

Step #1: If you have bowel issues and you're depressed, you should talk to your doctor about testing for celiac disease.

Step #2: If celiac disease is confirmed, eat a gluten-free diet, take probiotics, and have comprehensive testing for nutritional deficiencies, which are common in celiac disease (and could be contributing to depression).

Step #3: Correct any deficiencies with targeted nutritional supplementation.

Candida albicans

Step #1: If you have a chronic fungal infection, take the probiotic supplement *Saccharomyces boulardii*.

   Dosage: five billion CFU, three times a day.

Step #2: Eat more antifungal foods and spices, like garlic extract and gingerroot.

Step #3: Minimize sugar.

Step #4: Take the supplement caprylic acid, ideally in combination with thymol and carvacrol, two components of oregano oil.

   Dosage: Follow the recommendation on the label.

Step #5: Talk to your physician about taking Nystatin, an antifungal drug.

Step #6: If you have a persistent, localized fungal infection, like athlete's foot, talk to your doctor about the best topical antifungal for you.

CHAPTER 12

The Care and Feeding of Your Hormones

> Test and treat for hormonal imbalances—
> a common but overlooked cause of depression.

You know about your *circulatory system*—with the heart at its beating core, circulating blood throughout your body. And your *immune system*, with cellular watchguards like macrophages looking for foreign invaders. And your *respiratory system*, inhaling oxygen and exhaling carbon dioxide. And your *digestive system*, breaking down foods into absorbable components and getting rid of the rest.

But you're probably a little less familiar with the workings of your *endocrine system*, the hormone-secreting glands of the body like the thyroid gland and the adrenal glands. You may not know the names of those glands, or the hormones they manufacture, or the functions those hormones perform. So, what does your endocrine system do, exactly?

Well, think of your hormones as chemical messengers, traveling throughout the body via the bloodstream, telling cells and organs what to do. Some hormones control growth. Others control your metabolism, including your heart rate, speed of digestion, and body temperature. And all your hormones function via *feedback*: if you're overheated, for example, they work like a thermostat, telling the cooling mechanisms of the body (like sweating) to get into action.

This feedback mechanism sometimes works like a set of dominoes, with one hormone telling another hormone to get busy, and *that* hormone issuing its own set of instructions.

If you're depressed and want to feel good again, there are two essential facts about your endocrine system and your hormones that you need to know:

1) Hormones can affect mood—and hormone imbalances are a common but often-overlooked factor in depression.

2) If you're being treated for depression, your doctor should check for levels of key hormones—and correct imbalances.

Now, I have a confession to make: I'm *not* an endocrinologist, a doctor who specializes in hormones. Yes, I test my patients for hormonal imbalances—particularly thyroid hormones, arguably the most influential hormones in depression. But if the tests reveal imbalances, I refer my patient to an endocrinologist, a specialist in the hormone-generating endocrine system. So, this chapter will have a slightly different approach than the other chapters in the book. It will *not* present the step-by-step approach that I typically implement with patients. It *will* inform you about the hormones involved in depression, so you can work with a doctor to find and fix imbalances.

Thyroid Hormones: Managing Your Metabolic Factory

The thyroid is a small, butterfly-shaped gland that wraps around the voice box (larynx) and windpipe (trachea). The hormones it produces control metabolism—the speed of key functions like heart rate and digestion.

The thyroid communicates with the rest of the body via two main hormones: thyroxine (T4) and triiodothyronine (T3). But communication breaks down when levels of one or both of these hormones are too low (hypothyroidism) or too high (hyperthyroidism).

Low levels are the most common problem, and they generate a wide range of possible symptoms, including depression, fatigue, and anxiety. Other common symptoms include:

- memory and concentration problems;

- low sex drive;

- constipation;

- high cholesterol;

- gum disease;

- obesity;

- low blood sugar (hypoglycemia);

- muscle aches and pains;

- dry skin;

- acne;

- eczema;

- hair loss;

- recurrent infections;

- irregular menstrual periods;

- severe premenstrual syndrome;

- ovarian cysts;

- endometriosis;

- fluid retention;

- intolerance to cold; and/or

- lower sweat production.

Inaccurate testing, ineffective treatment

You'd think that detecting and treating low levels of thyroid hormones would be simple and straightforward: Check the level, correct the level.

Unfortunately—for the estimated 13 percent of Americans with low levels, nine out of ten of them women—it's neither simple nor straight-forward.

Even when doctors check for thyroid hormones—and that's nowhere near often enough—the main test they use isn't very accurate. A conventional doctor who suspects a thyroid problem usually does *not* check for levels of free T3 and free T4 in the blood. (The "free" portion is the biologically active portion.) Instead, they use a blood test called the Thyroid-Stimulating Hormone (TSH) Test. Here's where things get a little bit complicated, but bear with me, because this info could be crucial as you figure out with your health care provider how to find and fix an imbalance in thyroid hormones.

TSH isn't a thyroid hormone—it's released by the pituitary gland in the brain, which uses TSH to tell the thyroid gland the body needs more T3 and T4. Basically, this blood test doesn't answer the question, "Are your levels of thyroid hormones low?" Instead, it answers the question, "How much thyroid hormone does the pituitary gland think the body needs?" And many doctors presume that if the TSH level is high, it means there are many requests for thyroid hormones, which in turn means the thyroid is not making enough hormones. In other words, a person with a *high* TSH has *low* thyroid hormone production, or hypothyroidism.

On the other hand, if TSH levels are low, many doctors think it must mean the cells, tissues, and organs aren't requesting much thyroid hormone—not even routine amounts. This implies an overactive thyroid, or hyperthyroidism.

And if TSH levels are balanced (0.4 to 4.5 milli-international units per liter, or mIU/L), everything is A-OK with the thyroid.

To recap: A high TSH means the thyroid is pumping out too little hormone; a low TSH means too much; and a balanced TSH means the thyroid is working just right. But there are plenty of problems with relying on this test as the sole marker of thyroid health.

The usefulness of the TSH test is based on the assumption that the pituitary always requests the correct amount of thyroid hormone—an assumption that has no scientific evidence supporting it. Suppose, for example, that the pituitary itself is off-kilter and requests too little or too much hormone. Why assume when testing the health of the thyroid that the pituitary is working fine? And that's not the only problem with the test.

How much TSH is *really* normal and healthy? The TSH Test has been popular since the 1960s, but there is no conclusive scientific evidence demonstrating a healthy range. In fact, the normal range has been repeatedly changed over the years.

Many integrative functional doctors, for example, think a TSH level of more than 2.5 (well within the so-called "normal" range) indicates a sluggish thyroid. In fact, I've seen many patients with "normal" TSH who clearly had hypothyroidism.

Bottom line: Many people with a thyroid problem might be misdiagnosed on the basis of a TSH Test—that is, they're told they *don't* have an under- or overactive thyroid, when in fact they do! In my clinical experience, that includes many people with depression.

The best way to determine thyroid problems linked to depression: measure free T3 and free T4 levels. If levels are low, your doctor may choose to treat them with Synthroid (levothyroxine) for T4 and/or Cytomel (liothyronine) for T3, or natural desiccated thyroid (NDT), a product that supplies both T3 and T4. And treatment may be necessary even when levels are within the range considered "normal." That's because so-called *subclinical* levels of low thyroid hormones—levels that are in the lower range of normal—also can cause depression.

Scientific support

I'm hardly the first doctor to link low levels of thyroid hormones to depression. In fact, the first studies using thyroid hormones to treat depression were conducted in the 1960s. And there are plenty of more recent studies linking hypothyroidism and depression. For example:

Low-normal T4 = higher risk of depression. In a five-year study published in the July 20, 2023, issue of the *Journal of the Endocrine Society*, Japanese researchers looked at data from nearly sixty-seven thousand people with so-called "normal" thyroid function. They found that those with "low-normal" T4 had a 15 to 24 percent higher risk of major depression.[1]

Physical symptoms of depression "remarkably improved." In a study published in *Endocrine Research* in 2015, sixty people with subclinical hypothyroidism were given either levothyroxine (T4) or a placebo for twelve weeks. In those taking levothyroxine, depression scores dropped by 26 percent—with no drop in those taking the placebo. In addition, some of the physical symptoms of depression "remarkably improved," said the researchers—with better sleep, less fatigue, better appetite, and fewer aches and pains.[2]

Increasing the T4 dose decreases depression. Korean researchers increased the "baseline dose" of levothyroxine in twenty-four people being treated for hypothyroidism—and lowered depression levels by 21 percent. Treatment with levothyroxine "might be an ancillary [additional] treatment for depression," concluded the researchers in the August 2020 issue of *Clinical Endocrinology*.[3]

Treating with T4 and T3 works better. In a study by Polish researchers, published in the September 2018 issue of *Current Medical Research and Opinion*, adding T3 treatment (liothyronine) to standard T4 treatment (levothyroxine) in premenopausal women with hypothyroidism decreased depression scores (and increased sexual desire).[4]

Women: Boost your mood—and protect your heart. Treating people with subclinical hypothyroidism and depression doesn't only boost mood—it also protects against heart disease. In a Chinese study, published in the July 4, 2023, issue of *Frontiers in Psychiatry*, researchers looked at 1,744 women with depression—and found that those with depression *and* subclinical hypothyroidism had a much higher risk of cardiovascular disease than depressed women with normal thyroids. "The increased cardiovascular disease risk in female depressed patients with subclinical hypothyroidism requires more attention from researchers and clinicians," concluded the researchers.[5]

Mayo Clinic confirms: Thyroid imbalance and depression are linked. In a study published in the July 2023 issue of *Mayo Clinical Proceedings*, researchers looked at data from twenty-nine thousand people—and found that imbalanced thyroid hormone levels increased the risk of depression by 37 percent.[6]

Three steps

Based on the scientific evidence, I think everyone who is being evaluated or treated for depression should have their thyroid function tested. And that means more than the TSH Test, as I've just discussed. Try to find a doctor who takes a functional approach to depression—and discuss this three-step approach:

1. Evaluate for all symptoms of thyroid dysfunction, as I listed them above. The more symptoms you have, the more likely your thyroid hormones are low.

2. Measure your basal body temperature at the same time of day, over several days, ideally before getting out of bed in the morning. You might have a temperature lower than 98.6°F, which is more evidence that you have hypothyroidism.

3. Test levels of free T3, free T4, and TSH.

I can't overstate the importance of thyroid testing and treatment in depression. It's crucial to find out if your thyroid is underactive—and to work with a doctor to fix the problem if it's discovered.

Thyroid antibodies

In some cases, low thyroid functioning is caused by an autoimmune disease: Hashimoto's thyroiditis, in which the immune system attacks the thyroid as if it were a foreign invader, unbalancing hormones. This produces thyroid peroxidase (TPO) antibodies and antithyroglobulin (ATG) antibodies, a sure sign that your thyroid is under attack. It's important that you are tested not only for thyroid hormone levels, but also for TPO antibodies. The optimal range is less than 2 international units per milliliter (IU/mL) for TPO and less than 10 IU/mL for ATG antibodies.

Iodine: helping out the thyroid

The trace mineral iodine is a must for the creation of thyroid hormones—and a deficiency of iodine can cause thyroid problems. (However, too *much* iodine can hurt your thyroid.) You might think that iodine deficiency has become a rarity because of the widespread use of iodized salt. But not all salt *is* iodized, with only 50 percent of Americans using the product regularly—and one in nine Americans having low blood levels of iodine. Even with iodized salt, many people still need supplemental iodine. Consider testing blood levels to see if you're one of them.

Toxins and the thyroid

The thyroid gland is particularly vulnerable to environmental toxins—the approximately eighty thousand synthetic chemicals that are found in air, water, food, and consumer products. For example, polychlorinated biphenyls (PCBs)—a designation that includes more than two hundred similar chemicals—are found literally everywhere on earth, including the cells of your body. The problem: These chemicals (and others) can interact with and disrupt normal thyroid function.

Protect your thyroid by doing your best to minimize exposure to toxic chemicals. Eat organic when you can. Use all-natural cleaning products, like white vinegar. And for food storage, forego the plastic, and favor glass, ceramic, or stable metals like stainless steel.

Sex Hormones:
The Ups and Downs

The sex hormones testosterone, estrogen, and progesterone can play a role in depression.

Testosterone: One in five older men need more

Testosterone is the hormone that gives men upper-body strength, a deep voice, a beard—and a sex drive to match. It's also responsible for a wide variety of positive health effects, including making the thousands of proteins that regulate cellular health, ensuring healthy muscles and bones, and maintaining the receptors for the neurotransmitter serotonin.

But testosterone levels decline with age—falling by an average 1.6 percent per year after a man's twenties, with one in five men over the age of sixty below the normal range. Symptoms of low testosterone can include fatigue, low libido, decreased strength, high blood pressure, the loss of muscle, and the accumulation of fat. And in men, low testosterone can also cause depression. The evidence:

Twenty-seven studies show—testosterone treatment also treats depression. In a meta-analysis of twenty-seven studies involving 1,890 men, European researchers found that "testosterone treatment appears to be effective and efficacious in reducing depressive symptoms in men." In fact, the men taking the testosterone had more than double the reduction in symptoms compared to men taking a placebo—230 percent, to be exact. The results were reported in the January 2019 issue of *JAMA Psychiatry*.[7]

If your testosterone levels are low, see an endocrinologist or another provider who specializes in hormonal treatment for possible testosterone replacement therapy. The provider can rule out other causes of low testosterone, like a pituitary gland tumor or a chronic disease. And they can monitor the effects of the therapy, including possible side effects like headaches, gum pain, breast growth, nausea, and dizziness, and adjust the dose accordingly.

Estrogen and progesterone: Balance is a must

Estrogen (a group of hormones, including estradiol, estrone, and estriol) and progesterone are two hormones that play a vital role in a woman's reproductive system, but also affect the immune system, heart, bones, skin, and many other parts of the body—including the brain.

These hormones and mood are closely linked. Many women experience mood changes (including depression) during their menstrual cycle, after giving birth, and during perimenopause and menopause.

But hormonal influences on mood are much more complex in women than they are in men, and there is no dependable formula for testing and treatment like, "More estrogen = less depression." The key is *balancing* estrogen and progesterone, a challenging process that should be done under the supervision of an endocrinologist or another provider who specializes in hormone assessment and treatment.

Pregnenolone:
The "Mother Hormone"

Pregnenolone is sometimes called the "mother hormone" because it's a precursor to many other hormones in the body, including testosterone, estrogen, progesterone, and dehydroepiandrosterone (DHEA), which I'll talk about in a moment.

Produced in the adrenal glands from cholesterol, pregnenolone can cross the blood-brain barrier, functioning as a so-called *neurosteroid*. And as a neurosteroid, it plays an important role in regulating mood, memory, and cognitive function. Clinicians have used pregnenolone to:

- reduce the symptoms of depression and anxiety;

- stabilize mood swings;

- boost energy and motivation;

- combat mental and physical fatigue;

- enhance thinking and decision-making;

- improve memory and learning capacity;

- focus attention, and improve mental clarity; and

- clear up brain fog and stop cognitive decline.

There are a few studies on pregnenolone and depression. Two examples:

Bipolar depression: 61 percent in remission. Scientists from the Department of Psychiatry at Duke University Medical Center and several other institutions conducted a study on pregnenolone as an addition to drug treatment for bipolar depression. Sixty-one percent of those taking the hormone went into remission—compared to 37 percent of those taking a placebo. "Pregnenolone may improve depressive symptoms in patients with BPD and can be safely administered," wrote the researchers in *Neuropsychopharmacology*.[8]

Depression and substance abuse: Pregnenolone helps. Psychiatrists at the University of Texas studied seventy people with a "dual diagnosis"—major depressive disorder (MDD) *and* a history of substance abuse. The seventy participants took either 100 mg of daily pregnenolone or a placebo for eight weeks. Those taking the hormone had a significant reduction in depressive symptoms compared to those taking the placebo. Pregnenolone was safe and well tolerated, wrote the researchers in *Psychiatry Research*.[9]

If you and your doctor decide on treatment with pregnenolone, keep the following in mind:

Have a doctor order a blood test to determine your levels of pregnenolone.

Start with a low dose (10 to 50 mg), and increase gradually, to no more than 100 mg.

Morning intake is better than later in the day; pregnenolone can keep you awake.

As with all hormones, you should receive regular monitoring, to make sure levels are stable.

Possible side effects include headaches, sleep disturbances, anxiety (at higher levels), acne or other skin changes, and changes in the levels of other hormones. If you experience side effects, reduce pregnenolone or discontinue it.

If you have a hormone-sensitive condition, like premenstrual dysphoric disorder—severe mood swings associated with the menstrual cycle—pregnenolone may not be for you.

The Adrenal Glands and DHEA

The adrenal glands produce adrenaline (epinephrine), the hormone that fuels the fight-or-flight response—speeding up heart rate, spiking blood pressure, tensing muscles, expanding airways, pumping out blood sugar, increasing strength and energy, and dulling pain. That's one powerful hormone!

But there's another adrenal hormone that's far more abundant than adrenaline, and plays a big role in everyday life and health: DHEA (dehydroepiandrosterone).

Without DHEA, it's harder for your body to produce the sex hormones testosterone or estrogen. DHEA also plays a role in the strength of the immune system, in levels of energy and fatigue, and in maintaining healthy bones. And—as you've probably guessed by its inclusion in this chapter—DHEA influences mood. A few scientific studies illustrate the point:

Lower DHEA levels, more recurrent depression. German researchers measured salivary levels of several hormones over a three-day period in two groups of people with MDD—one group who was having their first depressive episode; and one group who had recurrent episodes. The only hormone that was uniquely low in the recurrent group was DHEA. "DHEA could represent a significant biomarker of major depressive disorder progression," wrote the researchers in the May 2023 issue of *Journal of Psychiatric Research*. And, they say, DHEA could be used in the "individualized treatment" of MDD—particularly to help a depressed person handle stress better.[10]

In a similar study, published in the September 2015 issue of *Psychoneuroendocrinology*, Dutch researchers found that people with lower morning levels of DHEA were more likely to have recurrent episodes of depression.[11]

Depressed people produce less DHEA. Chinese scientists looked at levels of DHEA and DHEA-S (the storage form of the hormone) in thirty-eight depressed people and forty-three people without depression who took a psychological test designed to create acute stress. The depressed people produced much lower levels of DHEA and DHEA-S during the test. These results were published in the June 2017 issue of the *Journal of Affective Disorders*.[12]

Seventy-two percent improvement with DHEA. In a small study from researchers at the University of California, San Francisco, six middle-aged and elderly people with major depression and low levels of DHEA or DHEA-S were given 30 to 90 mg of DHEA daily for four weeks—a dose intended to boost blood levels to levels seen in young people. All of the patients had an improvement in depressive symptoms, and in memory—improvements that vanished after the hormone was discontinued. In the case of a "treatment-resistant" woman who received DHEA during the study and for the next six months, depressive symptoms improved by 72 percent, and memory improved by 63 percent.

"DHEA may have antidepressant effects," concluded the researchers in the February 1997 issue of *Biological Psychiatry*.[13]

Twenty-two studies conclude: DHEA works. When Brazilian researchers analyzed data from twenty-two studies on depression and DHEA, they came to a simple conclusion: "Significant improvements related to the use of DHEA in patients with depression were observed." (They also saw improvements in depression in patients with schizophrenia, anorexia, and HIV.)[14]

If you're being evaluated or treated for depression, your doctor should measure DHEA.

CHAPTER 13

Inner Strengths, Outer Connections

> Interventions like cognitive behavioral therapy can assist you in self-understanding and self-care.

ere is the most important fact about therapy and depression: Therapy works.

Also called "talk therapy" or "counseling," therapy involves meeting regularly with a psychologist, psychiatrist, or other trained mental health professional to identify and treat your mental health conditions and emotional challenges.

Three out of four people who enter therapy show some benefit from it, according to the American Psychiatric Association. And that includes depressed people. A study from the World Health Organization looked at a database that includes all of the clinical trials testing therapy for depression from the past sixteen years. The researchers' conclusion:

Therapy "can contribute considerably to a reduction of the disease burden of depression."[1]

Yes, it's true that this book presents a biology-based plan for treating depression. But it's also true that depression is an amalgam of biology *and* psychology. And no treatment is truly integrative if it doesn't address the body and the mind.

Why Therapy Works

There are many ways therapy can help you if you're depressed.

Understanding the causes. A trained therapist can help you identify the factors that are contributing to your depression, like traumas from the past or thought patterns in the present. This increased self-awareness helps you feel more in control, less helpless—and less depressed.

Changing thoughts and beliefs. Many forms of therapy—including cognitive behavioiral therapy (CBT), the most-studied therapy for depression—focus on identifying negative thought patterns and beliefs. By recognizing and altering these self-defeating thoughts and beliefs, you can reduce depressive symptoms—particularly when you're under stress.

Getting active. CBT and other therapies teach the techniques of "behavioral activation"—intentionally engaging in enjoyable and fulfilling activities, even if you're not motivated to do so. This behavioral approach helps overcome the apathy, inactivity, and withdrawal that are common in depression.

Managing emotions. Many forms of therapy teach you strategies for managing your emotions—healthier ways to cope with sadness, anxiety, and anger. These strategies can reduce the intensity and duration of depressive episodes.

Solving practical problems. When you're depressed, you feel overwhelmed by the challenges of daily life. Therapy can help you develop problem-solving skills to address real-life issues that are contributing to your depression.

Improving relationships. Therapy can address difficulties in your interpersonal relationships—difficulties that are often a cause and a consequence of depression. Plus, enhancing social support reduces feelings of isolation.

Enhancing self-care. A therapist can work with you to establish a self-care routine that includes healthier lifestyle choices, like eating whole foods, exercising regularly, getting enough sleep, and managing stress.

Providing support. A therapist provides you with a supportive, safe environment to express your thoughts and feelings, without judgment. When you feel understood, you feel less lonely.

Preventing relapse. Therapy can help you develop strategies to minimize the risk of future depressive episodes. Perhaps the most important of those strategies: recognizing and addressing the early warning signs of depression, like anxiety, sadness, irritability, fatigue, or insomnia.

Now that you know *why* therapy works, let's take a closer look at the most effective therapy for depression: CBT.

Cognitive Behavioral Therapy: New Thoughts, New Actions

Cognitive behavioral therapy (CBT) is the most-researched therapy for depression—and one of the most effective. A meta-analysis of 409 studies on CBT for depression, involving nearly fifty-three thousand people, was published in the February 2023 issue of *World Psychiatry*.[2] The research concluded that CBT:

- has "moderate to large effects" in reducing depressive symptoms;

- is significantly more effective than other therapies;

- is more effective than medication, particularly in the long term (six to twelve months after therapy); and

- is effective in an unguided self-help format, like using a book or taking an online course.

CBT typically consists of twelve to twenty sessions of fifty minutes each (the length of most therapy sessions). The goal of CBT is to reduce negative or unhelpful thoughts, actions, attitudes, and beliefs that are common in people with depression. In CBT, you actively *challenge* those depressive patterns—and create new, positive patterns. The process usually involves:

Assessment. You and the therapist identify your specific symptoms of depression, along with their duration and severity.

Education. The therapist educates you about the CBT approach: how thoughts, emotions, and behaviors are interconnected; and how negative thought patterns can contribute to and worsen depressive symptoms.

Setting goals. You and your therapist set specific and achievable treatment goals for reducing symptoms. These goals are monitored throughout therapy, with adjustments in strategy to address challenges and promote improvement.

Identifying negative thought patterns. You learn to identify the negative thoughts that contribute to your depression. CBT calls these thoughts "cognitive distortions" or "thinking errors"—irrational or exaggerated beliefs about yourself, others, or the future. An example: "I'm a failure—I'll never do anything right." One way to identify thinking errors is with "thought journaling"—keeping a journal to write down and explore your thoughts, emotions, and behaviors.

Challenging and restructuring thoughts. Once you recognize negative thought patterns, you can change them—by challenging their validity and accuracy, and by "reframing" and "restructuring" negative thoughts into more balanced, rational thoughts.

Behavioral activation. You identify activities that bring you a sense of pleasure, achievement, and connection with others—and you work with your therapist to set goals relative to increasing those activities (and rewarding yourself when you do so). This is called *activity scheduling*.

Problem-solving skills. CBT sessions teach you to identify problems, generate solutions—and implement strategies to put the solutions into place.

Coping skills. These daily skills help you manage depression and prevent relapse. They include techniques for relaxation, stress management, and handling negative emotions.

Homework and practice. Between sessions, you're assigned "homework" to practice the skills and techniques you learned in therapy.

Relapse prevention. Toward the end of CBT treatment, you work with your therapist to develop a plan for preventing relapse.

There are several variations of CBT available. They include:

- **Acceptance and Commitment Therapy**, which encourages acceptance of thoughts and feelings, and commitment to behavioral change;

Thinking Errors in Depression

According to cognitive behavioral therapy, there are ten common thinking errors in depression:

1) **Mind reading.** Assuming others are thinking negatively about you.

2) **Catastrophizing.** Making negative predictions about the future based on little or no evidence.

3) **All-or-nothing thinking.** Viewing something as either-or, without considering the full spectrum and range of possible outcomes.

4) **Emotional reasoning.** Believing something to be true based on emotional responses rather than objective evidence.

5) **Labeling.** Classifying yourself negatively after an adverse event.

6) **Mental filtering.** Focusing on negative information and devaluing positive information.

7) **Overgeneralization.** Assuming that when one bad thing happens more bad things will happen.

8) **Personalization.** Assuming you're the cause of a negative event.

9) **"Should" statements.** Thinking things "should" or must be a certain way.

10) **Minimizing or disqualifying the positive.** Acknowledging but dismissing or discounting positive things that have happened.

CBT teaches methods to reduce the power of thinking errors, like keeping a "thought log"—you write down and consider your thinking errors and learn to think more objectively.

- **Dialectical Behavioral Therapy**, which was initially developed to treat people with frequent suicidal thoughts; and

- **Rational Emotive Behavior Therapy**, which uses the desire to feel happy to guide people with depression in the process of changing thoughts and behavior.

Internet-based CBT

There are numerous studies proving the efficacy of internet-based CBT for depression—for homebound older adults; for people with chronic back pain; delivered as self-help, without a therapist; for people with suicidal ideation; and many other situations.

Other Types of Therapy

There are many other types of therapy that are used to help resolve depression and prevent a relapse, and that have proven their efficacy in clinical studies.

They include:

Narrative Therapy. This therapy is based on the understanding that you organize your life experiences in narrative form—a story. By exploring the stories that reflect your depression, the therapist helps you generate alternative stories to rewrite your life's narrative.

Psychodynamic Therapy. Akin to classic Freudian analysis, this therapy offers an intense exploration of your feelings, and also delves deeply into the past, offering you the opportunity to resolve early psychological trauma.

Interpersonal Therapy. This therapy—intended to be completed in twelve to sixteen weeks—focuses on resolving interpersonal relationships and reducing depressive symptoms.

Humanistic Therapy. This therapy aims at "self-actualization"—the expression of your full potential. In the process of this therapy, you explore your feelings, find meaning in life, and develop a strong and positive sense of self.

Find a Therapist You Trust

Perhaps the most important factor in therapy is the therapist.

To find a therapist, ask a family member, friend, or your health care provider for a recommendation—this almost always works better than a random search. Often, your health care provider will be aware of therapists in your area because the provider's patients tell them about therapists they like.

In your first appointment, be direct. Tell the therapist exactly what you're looking to achieve in therapy.

Most importantly, find a therapist you feel you can *trust.*

If you trust your therapist, you're more likely to enter into the process of therapy with an open mind and an open heart.

And if interpersonal difficulties have been a factor in depression, relating to a trusted therapist who doesn't react to you in the sometimes dysfunctional ways of family members (spouse, children, parents, etc.) can help you overcome your sadness.

In my clinical practice, I have observed that some depressed patients—often busy, successful professionals—arrive at my office alone, and have been secretive about their struggles with depression. Depression is often marked by this kind of social withdrawal and inertia. Talking to a trusted therapist can restore your ability to relate—and to act.

Finally, a trusted therapist can help you *be yourself.*

As you search for a therapist, find someone who is supportive of your needs, and respects you as an individual. A good therapist doesn't think that there is only one therapy that is the answer for everyone. A good therapist recognizes and appreciates that everyone is *unique*—and finds the therapy and approach that *you* respond to.

Psychedelic Therapy for Depression

Is It for You?

The last decade has seen a surge of scientific interest in the therapeutic powers of *psychedelics*—consciousness-altering drugs like psilocybin, ketamine, LSD, mescaline, ayahuasca, and MDMA. And by surge, I do mean *surge*.

Currently, there are more than 350 government-approved clinical trials on ketamine for depression, and more than eighty on psilocybin for depression. In other words, there's a *lot* of interest.

In the short term, psychedelics work by activating the same neurotransmitter targeted by antidepressants: serotonin, the brain chemical that regulates functions like mood, emotions, sleep, appetite, and sex drive. Psychedelics attach to the 2A receptor for serotonin, the first step in a series of many that produces an array of psychological effects. (Ketamine—a so-called "non-classic" psychedelic—affects the transmission of the neurotransmitter glutamate.)

The result? Psychedelics activate parts of the brain that are typically dormant. They also quiet parts of the brain that are typically active, like the prefrontal cortex, which regulates thinking.

Not only are different areas energized or subdued—the way different parts of the brain communicate with one another is also changed. Dramatically.

There is a huge uptick in what researchers call "global connectivity"—parts of the brain that don't normally communicate with each other start to interact.

Think of it this way, says Matthew Johnson, PhD (author of more than fifty scientific papers on psychedelics, former Susan Hill Ward Professor of Psychedelics and Consciousness at the Johns Hopkins University School of Medicine, and currently a senior researcher for the Center of Excellence for Psilocybin Research and Treatment at Sheppard Pratt's Institute for Advanced Diagnostics and Therapeutics):

"Normally, 'local networks' in the brain mostly communicate with their next-door neighbors. When you take a psychedelic, those same networks communicate less with the neighbors and more with the people across town."

These brain changes, says Dr. Johnson, typically produce what could be called a "mystical experience," which can include: a positive mood; a sense of wholeness and connection with oneself and with the outside world; a sense of direct knowledge of the nature of reality; a sense of everything being sacred or holy; transcendence of time and space; and a sense of ineffability, or the fact that reality is beyond definition and language.

And this type of experience can have positive therapeutic effects, including relieving depression—even depression after a terminal diagnosis, like fourth-stage cancer.

"A mystical experience while taking a psychedelic can grant a new perspective on life and self that allows a person to have a fundamental psychological resolution of their condition or disorder," says Dr. Johnson.

Research supports this statement. Two examples among many:

Fifty-eight percent of major depression in remission—with psilocybin. In a study in the *Journal of Pharmacology*, published in February 2022, psilocybin was tested on twenty-seven people with major depressive disorder (MDD). Each person received two doses of psilocybin with supportive psychotherapy. After a year, three out of four patients had more than a 50 percent reduction in depression and 58 percent had complete remission. The experience of "personal meaning, spiritual experience, and mystical experience" during the psychedelic session predicted the subsequent level of well-being.[3]

Thirty percent reduction in symptoms—with psilocybin. In a study published in *Psychiatry Research* in February 2025, an international team of scientists analyzed three studies on psilocybin and MDD, involving 389 people. After two weeks, those who took a 25 milligram (mg) dose of psilocybin had a 30 percent reduction in depressive symptoms. This analysis, wrote the researchers, "supports psilocybin's efficacy in treating major depressive disorder."[4]   *(continued)*

Thirty percent increase in rates of remission—with ketamine. In a study published in the *Journal of Psychiatric Research* in December 2024, researchers analyzed results from nine studies involving 1,752 patients who had taken Spravato (esketamine), an FDA-approved, ketamine-derived nasal spray for treatment-resistant depression. Compared to placebo, 30 percent more people went into remission after using Spravato.[5]

And a July 1, 2024, study in the *Journal of Affective Disorders*, from the Department of Psychiatry at Yale University School of Medicine and several other institutions, analyzed twenty-one studies on ketamine and treatment-resistant depression, involving more than two thousand people. The researchers concluded the results on ketamine were "highly clinically meaningful in this difficult to treat disorder." In other words, where no other drug worked, ketamine is very likely to work![6]

But don't expect to see the word "psychedelic" on your psychiatrist's prescription pad anytime soon. As of this writing, Spravato is the only psychedelic currently approved by the FDA. (However, the FDA has also granted "breakthrough therapy designation" to a psilocybin-based drug—Cybin—for MDD, meaning if the Phase 3 clinical trial on the drug is positive, it will go quickly to market. In a Phase 2 trial of the drug, 75 percent of participants achieved remission, showing no signs of depression.[7])

Bottom line: Except for Spravato, the use of psychedelics is still illegal under federal law, except in government-approved clinical trials. While several cities and states have decriminalized psilocybin, these local laws don't cancel federal law.

What to do

So, what should you do if you want to avail yourself of psychedelic therapy?

Of course, you can talk to your doctor about Spravato, and whether or not it's right for you.

Along with that option, the only legal, safe way to use psychedelics is to participate in a clinical trial. Otherwise, you're risking your health and well-being. (For example, people with severe heart disease have died taking psilocybin.) To safely take a psychedelic, your experience should be legal; using a compound you can trust for purity and dose; with a medical screening beforehand; and psychological support during and after the experience.

How to find a clinical trial

To find a clinical trial, go to the database www.clinicaltrials .gov. Under "Condition or Disease," write "depression." Under "Intervention/treatment," write "psychedelic" or "psilocybin" or "ketamine," depending on your interest. Under "Status," check "Recruiting and not yet recruiting studies." Under "Condition or disease," enter "depression." Under "Other terms," use the word "psychedelic," or "ketamine," or "psilocybin," depending on your interest. When the site asks you to "Focus Your Search," with one of the options "Study Status," check "Recruiting" and "Not yet recruiting." You'll end up with a lot of options, which you can further refine by where you live, the distance you're willing to travel, etc. Alternatively, you can enter the word "psychedelic" in the "Other terms" field—and review the more than six hundred studies currently listed on the website.

CHAPTER 14

Lifestyle Healing

Here's how to build more health—and
a better mood—into your daily schedule.

As I was writing this chapter on lifestyle and depression, a study appeared in the journal *Nature Mental Health*—a study that confirmed everything I was planning to present in this chapter; a large, landmark study that advances and confirms our scientific understanding of the link between a healthy lifestyle and mood. Here are the practical details of this important research.

Reducing Depression Risk by 57 Percent— with a Healthier Lifestyle

Conducted by an international team of researchers, including scientists from Cambridge University in England, the nine-year study analyzed health data from nearly two hundred ninety thousand people, thirteen thousand of whom had depression.[1]

The analysis revealed an important fact: Lifestyle and depression *are* linked.

Specifically, the following seven factors *reduced* the risk of depression:

- Healthy sleep

- Healthy diet

- Regular physical activity

- Less sedentary behavior (sitting, reclining, or lying)

- Frequent social connection

- Moderate alcohol consumption

- Never smoking

Of all these factors, getting a restful night's sleep—between seven and nine hours a night—made the biggest difference, reducing the risk of depression (including single depressive episodes and treatment-resistant depression) by 22 percent.

Frequent social connection (spending more time with family, friends, and other people) reduced the risk of depression by 18 percent. But social connection was the *most* protective of the lifestyle factors against recurrent depressive disorder.

These two depression-reducing lifestyle factors were followed in importance by: never smoking (20 percent reduction); regular physical activity (14 percent); less sedentary behavior (13 percent); moderate alcohol consumption (11 percent); and healthy diet (6 percent).

The researchers looked at the data another way, dividing the participants into three groups, based on the number of healthy lifestyle factors they adhered to: 1) favorable lifestyle; 2) intermediate lifestyle; and 3) unfavorable lifestyle.

Those in the favorable lifestyle group (with five or more lifestyle factors in their favor) were *57 percent less likely to develop depression*, compared to those in the unfavorable group.

Those in the intermediate group were 41 percent less likely.

Lifestyle is more important than genetics

The researchers also compared lifestyle factors to genetic factors.

They made that comparison by examining the DNA of all the participants, and assigning each person a genetic risk score based on the number of genetic variants an individual carried that have a known link to the risk of depression. Those with the lowest level of genetic risk factors were 25 percent less likely to have developed depression compared to those with the highest. Which means that genes had a *much, much smaller impact* on depression than lifestyle!

The researchers also found that lifestyle could cut the risk of depression among people with a high, medium, or low genetic risk. Put another way: a healthier lifestyle can work for *everybody* in lowering the risk of depression, no matter their genetic risk.

One of the study researchers, Professor Barbara Sahakian, from the Department of Psychiatry at the University of Cambridge, explained it this way: "Although our DNA—the genetic hand we're dealt—can increase our risk of depression, we've shown that a healthy lifestyle is potentially more important."

Why does lifestyle work?

To answer this question, the researchers looked at several factors.

Brain volume. A bigger brain is typically a healthier brain, with more neurons and more neural connections. To see if there was a correlation between brain size and lifestyle, the researchers took MRI scans of thirty-three thousand of the study participants. They found a number of brain regions—the amygdala, hippocampus, pallidum, and thalamus—where a larger volume was linked to a healthier lifestyle.

Inflammation. Low-grade, chronic inflammation—specifically, brain inflammation, or neuroinflammation—is linked to depression. To test the link between inflammation and lifestyle, the researchers measured C-reactive protein (CRP), a biomarker of inflammation. People with an unfavorable lifestyle had higher levels of CRP.

Metabolic health. A healthy metabolism—when the body efficiently uses energy from food—is key to well-being, including mental well-being. To measure metabolism, researchers measured levels of triglycerides, a type of stored fat made from excess calories; higher levels are a sign of an unhealthy metabolism. People with an unfavorable lifestyle had higher levels of triglycerides.

Bottom line: "We're used to thinking of a healthy lifestyle as being important to our *physical* health," said Dr. Christelle Langley, another study researcher at the Department of Psychiatry at the University of Cambridge. "But lifestyle is just as important for our *mental* health." I agree!

Simple Ways to a Healthier Lifestyle

Creating a healthier lifestyle is a lot simpler than you might imagine. You only need to make a few, easy changes to change your lifestyle from unfavorable to favorable.

Healthy sleep

Here are two easy ways to sleep deeper most nights.

Stick to a schedule. Set a specific time for going to bed at night and getting up in the morning—and stick to it. (For example, 11:00 P.M. and 7:00 A.M.) This regular schedule will balance your body's sleep/wake cycle, or circadian rhythms—and balanced circadian rhythms are the foundation of a good night's sleep.

Wear blue-light filtering glasses at night. The blue light emitted by screens—smartphones, TVs, computers, laptops, tablets, gaming consoles—reduces the production of melatonin, the sleep-inducing hormone. If you can, minimize your use of screens two hours before your bedtime. But if that's not realistic—and for many of us, it's not—wear blue-light filtering glasses at night, putting them on right after dinner.

Social connection

There are many ways that good relationships with family and friends are good for you.

Family and friends can encourage you to see a doctor when you're

Is Keto for You?

The high-fat, low-carb ketogenic diet (keto) is all the rage as a therapeutic eating style, especially for brain-based illnesses like epilepsy, Alzheimer's, Parkinson's, traumatic brain injury, and migraine.

Metabolically, the diet shifts the body's primary energy source from glucose (blood sugar) to fat and ketones, a state known as ketosis.

The effectiveness of the diet is likely due to several factors, including:

- Lower levels of insulin and glucose (blood sugar)
- More efficient mitochondria, tiny energy factories in every brain cell
- Less inflammation and oxidative stress

Could the ketogenic diet help in depression? The scientific evidence is promising.

In a recent study in *Nutritional Neuroscience*, scientists reviewed all the research to date on the ketogenic diet for major depressive disorder and treatment-resistant depression. They found "significant impact" for keto and other carbohydrate-restricting diets, with reduced depressive symptoms, better mood, and fewer depressive episodes. The diet, they add, is safe and straightforward to implement.[2]

In a recent case report in *Frontiers in Nutrition*, three people with major depression and generalized anxiety went on a ketogenic diet for three to four months. After seven weeks, two of the three patients had *complete remission* from both depression and anxiety.[3]

And a study in *British Journal of Psychiatry Open* showed the diet was effective in treating bipolar disorder, improving mood and energy, and decreasing impulsivity and anxiety.[4]

I see the ketogenic diet as a potentially helpful tool in depression and other psychiatric illnesses. It's not for everybody. And it can be difficult to maintain. But for those who want to try it, it's an option that might make a big difference.

sick, or to eat a healthier diet, or to take other actions that protect your health.

Strong social relationships buffer the effects of stress—and stress increases the risk for depression.

Relationships provide a sense of purpose and meaning to life, a factor that many studies show protects health.

Here are several ways to improve the social relationships you have, and add more social relationships to your life.

Don't rely on social media networks for intimate connection. Unless relationships transcend the cyberworld, they are not truly supportive. To really reach out and connect, pick up the phone and talk to your family and friends. Even better, meet up for lunch, dinner, or another social occasion. And establish true connection by being honest about yourself, sharing both the good and bad about your life.

Find new friends. Although social networks may not increase intimacy, you can use the internet constructively to find new friends you can spend time with at in-person events.

Volunteer. This is one of the best ways for people to create new social networks.

Do activities in a social environment. Whether it's exercising at a gym, attending adult education classes, or joining a bird-watching group—look for enjoyable activities you can do with others.

Regular physical activity

A 2022 study in the *British Journal of Sports Medicine* looked at forty-one studies on depression and exercise, involving 2,264 participants—and found that exercise improved depressive symptoms up to 39 percent. The authors' conclusion: Exercise works in treating depression and depressive symptoms.[5]

Go for a walk. Among people who succeed in exercising regularly, the most common exercise is *walking*. It's not hard to see why. Walking is easy, inexpensive, immediate, and convenient—you just put on a comfortable pair of walking shoes, wear weather-appropriate clothing, and step out the door. Walking is also safe—you're at a very low risk of injury. And walking can be social—it's fun to do with friends.

Another plus: walking doesn't require a lot of time. You can walk just a little while—like five to ten minutes a day—and still get plenty of feel-better benefits. You say you can only walk one minute? Well, start there, and gradually build up, by one minute per day. A study published in *JAMA Psychiatry* in 2022 showed that going from *no* activity to *some* activity is very helpful in preventing and reversing depression.[6]

Alcoholism, Nutrition, and Depression

Alcohol use disorder (AUD)—commonly referred to as alcoholism—is a devastating disease, affecting nearly twenty-nine million Americans, or about one in ten people aged twelve and older.

Alcohol abuse causes deadly accidents (alcohol is the cause of 5 percent of all deaths), poor health (four of ten hospital beds in America are occupied by people with alcohol-related illnesses), ruined relationships, and a host of other problems.

Including depression.

People with AUD are twice as likely to suffer from depressive symptoms.

Alcohol itself is a depressant, of course. But there's an often-overlooked cause of depression in AUD: nutritional deficiencies. Malnutrition is *common* in alcoholics, with excessive alcohol use linked to low levels of the B vitamins thiamine, riboflavin, niacin, pyridoxine, folate, and B12; vitamins C, D, and E; omega-3 fatty acids; and lithium. (It's a little-known fact that Bill W., the founder of Alcoholics Anonymous—or AA—championed high-dose niacin therapy for AA members, noting that the treatment helped many AA members overcome chronic depression.)

Low levels of many of these nutrients—like folate, B12, vitamin D, omega-3s, and lithium—are strongly linked to depression. Nutritional deficiencies in alcoholism also directly cause imbalances in neurotransmitters that trigger depression.

Bottom line: If you or a loved one has AUD, it's crucial to be tested for nutritional deficiencies—and to use targeted nutritional supplementation to correct any deficiencies.

But if walking isn't for you, don't worry. *Any* regular physical activity improves mental health, even household chores and gardening. Just get moving!

Less sedentary behavior

Sedentary behavior is when you're awake—and sitting or reclining, rather than moving around. And research shows too much sitting or lying around is bad for you. In fact, a study published in the *Lancet* looked at health data from more than one million people—and found that sitting for more than eight hours a day is as bad for you as smoking.[7] Unfortunately, 25 percent of Americans spend eight to ten hours a day sitting, at work, school, and home, while driving, in restaurants, and in movie theaters—anywhere there's a chair or a couch.

Stand up. But reducing sedentary behavior is simple: Just stand up!

Research shows that regularly standing up while sitting reduces many of its health risks, including overweight, high blood pressure, and high blood sugar. A good goal: Stand up for one minute every thirty minutes, throughout your day and evening. Even better is standing up and moving around a little.

Moderate alcohol consumption

"Moderate alcohol consumption" doesn't mean that a little bit of drinking is good for you. That once-popular scientific theory has been pretty much debunked. It means that if you do drink regularly, you don't drink too much. What's too much?

Well, the most recent research shows that *any* alcohol is potentially damaging to your health, because alcohol damages your DNA, increasing the risk for cancer, heart disease, liver disease, and other chronic health problems.

But if you want to enjoy alcohol as part of your lifestyle, a good rule of thumb is moderation: a small amount, with meals, and with family and friends.

Let There Be Light

Another lifestyle change that can deal with depression is getting more light in your life—particularly very bright light, particularly in the morning.

Light therapy—also called phototherapy—involves using a light box, which emits light a lot brighter than that of ordinary indoor lighting. In a study published in *American Family Physician* in 2021, researchers looked at all the studies to date using light therapy. They found that using bright white light, particularly in the morning, for sessions lasting less than sixty minutes, had a positive impact on depressive symptoms.[8]

Light therapy probably works by restoring normal circadian rhythm, the body's internal clock that matches the sleep/wake cycle (and many other functions) to the hours of the day. Typically, people who are depressed have a disturbed circadian rhythm. Light therapy also regulates the production of melatonin, a hormone that influences mood and sleep—when you're exposed to bright light in the morning, you reduce the production of melatonin, enhancing mood and alertness.

Research points to a "dose" of 10,000 lux (lux is a measurement of brightness, and 10,000 lux is about twenty times brighter than usual indoor lighting), for thirty minutes to one hour, each morning. Sit about sixteen to twenty-four inches from the light box, with your eyes open, but not staring directly at the light.

Light therapy is particularly effective for seasonal depressive disorder (SAD) but can help any type of depression.

Generally, light therapy is safe, without side effects. Some people might experience mild eyestrain, headache, nausea, and irritability, but that typically subsides after a few sessions. However, light therapy is *not* recommended for bipolar disorder (it may increase mania), and it's not recommended for people taking meditations that increase light sensitivity, or for people with severe sensitivity to light.

Healthy diet

You can read all about a healthy diet in Chapter 11, on digestion. But the most important guidelines are very simple:

Minimize your intake of ultra-processed foods (UPFs). Those are foods stripped of most or all of their natural nutrients and fiber, with lots of sugar, fat, salt, and artificial ingredients added.

Maximize your intake of whole, unprocessed foods. One science-supported, healthy pattern of eating whole foods is a Mediterranean-style diet, rich in whole grains, green leafy vegetables, legumes, nuts, berries, fish, chicken, and olive oil.

Final thoughts

Over the years, I've seen how difficult it is for my patients to make and maintain lifestyle changes. The key is making *simple* changes, one at a time. Only after you've formed a reliable habit—a process that typically takes about six weeks of steady adherence to the change—do you make the next change. We're talking about the "style" of your *life*, not of the next week or two. Slow (*very* slow) but steady (*very* steady) wins the lifestyle race.

STEP-BY-STEP ACTION PLAN FOR

Lifestyle Healing

Use this practical, step-by-step summary to implement the therapeutic actions discussed in this chapter.

Step #1: Sleep deeper by setting a specific time for going to bed at night and getting up in the morning.

Step #2: Improve social relationships by not relying on social media for intimate connections and volunteering.

Step #3: Walk regularly, even five to ten minutes per day.

Step #4: If you're sitting for long periods of time, stand up for one minute every thirty minutes.

Step #5: Minimize your intake of UPFs and maximize your intake of whole, unprocessed foods.

Step #6: Don't smoke. If you do smoke, quit.

PART FOUR

A NEW APPROACH TO ANTIDEPRESSANTS

CHAPTER 15

The Integrative Approach to Antidepressants

More Benefit, Less Risk

> Taking an antidepressant *and* nutritional supplements can improve the effectiveness of medication and help prevent side effects like weight gain and low libido.

Would you like your antidepressant medication to work *better*—to do a better job of keeping depression at bay and brightening your mood; and to work without the extra baggage of side effects like weight gain and low libido?

If you would, you're hardly alone.

Fifty to 60 percent of patients with depression *do not* obtain what doctors call an "adequate response"—that is, real relief—following their first treatment with antidepressants. And 35 percent fail to respond to *four* trials of antidepressants. (For major depressive disorder, or MDD, a trial of antidepressants is typically six to nine months.)

Medicine labels this group of patients—the non-responding 35 percent—"treatment resistant."

As I discussed earlier, I dislike that term because it blames the *patient* for the failure of the *medication*.

So, if your antidepressant isn't working as well as you'd like, what are your options?

You could talk to your doctor about increasing the dose of your current medication. Or you could ask about switching medications. Or you and your doctor could try adding another medication to boost the efficacy of the antidepressant, like an atypical antipsychotic or a mood stabilizer.

There are nondrug approaches, too.

You could complement the medicine with therapy, like cognitive behavioral therapy (CBT). (I talk about this strategy in Chapter 13.) Or you could incorporate healthy changes into your lifestyle, changes that are linked to less depression, like regular exercise or eating fewer ultraprocessed foods (UPFs). (I discuss these strategies in Chapter 14.)

However, all of those possibilities—with or without medication—are often limited in their impact. My favored approach—the strategy that works *best* for my patients in improving the performance of antidepressants—is *nutritional augmentation.*

Simply put, augmentation means adding targeted nutritional and herbal supplements to your antidepressant regimen. This strategy works because these targeted supplements support the action of antidepressants: They balance and boost mood-improving neurotransmitters like serotonin, dopamine, and norepinephrine.

In this chapter, we'll take a look at the top augmentation supplements, one by one, starting with the trace mineral zinc. (For dosages, please see the chapter where the supplement is more fully discussed.)

Zinc

As you read in Chapter 7, zinc is key to a balanced, healthy brain and positive moods. In fact, some scientists say that zinc is a *biomarker* for depression: The lower your levels of zinc, the more likely you'll feel depressed.

In my clinical experience, zinc is one of the best ways to augment antidepressants. And scientific research on zinc and antidepressants mirrors what I see in my patients. For example:

Selective serotonin reuptake inhibitors (SSRIs) work better with

zinc. In a study in *Nutritional Neuroscience*, thirty-seven people with MDD who were taking an SSRI were divided into two groups: one group took a daily dose of zinc, and the other group took a placebo. After twelve weeks, those taking zinc had "significantly reduced" scores in a standard test for depression (Hamilton Depression Rating Scale, or HAM-D) compared to those taking the placebo. Their mood was better; they had less anxiety; they felt less guilt; they had less insomnia; they were more able to work and participate in other activities; etc. "Zinc supplementation in conjunction with antidepressant drugs might be beneficial for reducing depressive symptoms," concluded the researchers.[1]

Overcoming "treatment-resistant" depression—with zinc. A university-based team of Polish psychiatrists studied sixty people with major depression who were treatment resistant, dividing them into two groups. Both groups were treated with Tofranil (imipramine)—but one group got Tofranil and a daily dose of 25 milligrams (mg) of zinc. After twelve weeks, "zinc supplementation significantly reduced depression scores and facilitated the treatment outcome in antidepressant treatment resistant patients," concluded the researchers in the *Journal of Affective Disorders*. They pointed out that zinc augmented the "speed" and "efficacy" of the antidepressant—in other words, with the addition of zinc, the drug worked faster and better.[2]

Conclusion: Zinc works. A 2022 study in *Nutritional Neuroscience* analyzed results from many different studies on augmentation with zinc and came to this positive conclusion: There is "evidence for the efficacy of zinc . . . as an [addition] to antidepressant medication."[3]

Omega-3

Chapter 9 was all about the omega-3 fatty acids docosahexaenoic acid (DHA) and eicosapentaenoic acid (EPA) and their power to ease depression. They can also make antidepressants work better:

Omega-3 and antidepressants—working better together. Researchers in India studied 165 people with mild to moderate depression, dividing them into three groups. The first group took an antidepressant; the second group took an omega-3 supplement; and the third group took an antidepressant *and* an omega-3 supplement. At the end of the study, those taking the antidepressant and omega-3 combo had the lowest level of depressive symptoms. In other words, the drug and the supplement worked better than either the drug alone or the supplement alone.[4]

The worse the depression, the greater the power of omega-3 to augment antidepressants. Polish researchers studied twenty-one patients with severe, treatment-resistant depression—they hadn't responded to eight weeks of treatment with either Effexor (venlafaxine) or Paxil (paroxetine). The researchers added omega-3 to the treatment regimen—a daily dose of 2.2 grams (g) of EPA and 700 mg of DHA.

(The supplement also included 240 mg of gamma-linoleic acid from primrose oil and 40 mg of vitamin E.)[5]

After four weeks on omega-3, the study participants had a 63 percent reduction in depressive symptoms—meaning their average level of depression was reduced from severe to mild, a significant decrease.

The researchers also note that omega-3 was just as effective as drugs used to augment antidepressants in the treatment of bipolar disorder, like lithium carbonate and the anticonvulsant drug Lamictal (lamotrigine). And they pointed out that the more severe and chronic the depression, the better omega-3 performed. Additionally, they highlighted the fact that there were other, important health benefits from omega-3: lower levels of low-density lipoprotein (LDL) cholesterol and triglycerides, two heart-hurting blood fats; and higher levels of "good," or high-density lipoprotein (HDL) cholesterol. That's a very important finding, since depression is linked to a 64 percent higher risk of coronary artery disease, and a 59 percent higher risk of a heart attack or death from heart disease.

The higher your level of omega-3, the better your response to antidepressants. In an eight-week study published in May 2022, European researchers looked at sixty people with severe depression who were taking antidepressants, dividing them into two groups: responders (the medication *was* working); and nonresponders (the medication *wasn't* working). They found that those with the lowest blood levels of omega-3 had the most severe depression. They also found that those with the lowest blood levels of omega-3 were far more likely to be nonresponders. Levels of omega-3 fatty acids predict response to antidepressants, concluded the researchers in the journal *Depression and Anxiety*. Omega-3, they wrote, is a new "tool for the management of unresponsive depression patients"—in other words, if someone isn't responding to antidepressant therapy, give them an omega-3 supplement![6]

Improved: Depression, anxiety, insomnia, uncertainty, and emotional control. Researchers from Switzerland studied fifty depressed people who were being treated with Zoloft (sertraline)—and added either an omega-3 supplement or a placebo to their regimen. After twelve weeks, the people taking omega-3 had:

- fewer symptoms of depression;

- less disturbance from anxiety;

- more tolerance of uncertainty;

- better sleep; and

- better regulation and control of emotions.

The study was published in the December 2018 issue of the *Journal of Psychiatric Research*.[7]

Achieving remission—by adding DHA. Twenty-eight treatment-resistant patients with mild to moderate depression were given a daily dose of either 260 or 520 mg of DHA to augment their antidepressant regimen. After eight weeks, more than half the patients had over a 50 percent reduction in their depression scores—and 45 percent were in complete remission. The results were reported in the April 2018 issue of *Nutritional Neuroscience*.[8]

Stopping depression after a heart attack—with an antidepressant *and* omega-3. About 20 percent of people who have a heart attack develop depression afterward. Researchers in Germany studied more than two thousand people after their heart attacks, publishing their results in the *Journal of Clinical Psychiatry*. Those who took an antidepressant *and* a daily omega-3 supplement had a "clinically relevant antidepressant effect"—but those who took *only* an antidepressant, or *only* an omega-3 supplement, saw no such effect. (The omega-3 supplement used in the study delivered a daily dose of 460 mg EPA and 380 mg DHA.)[9]

Folate

I discuss supplementing the diet with the B-vitamin folate in Chapter 6—with a focus on L-methylfolate (LMF), the biologically active form of the vitamin, and the only form that crosses the blood-brain barrier. Research shows LMF is key in helping antidepressants work.

LMF boosts the effectiveness of antidepressants.

Researchers from the University of South Carolina School of Medicine and the University of North Carolina, Chapel Hill, analyzed four studies that looked at the use of antidepressants *and* LMF to treat MDD. "These studies," they wrote in the May 9, 2023, issue of the *Primary Care Companion for CNS Disorders*, "support the use of LMF as an adjunctive [additional] treatment in patients with major depressive disorder not responding to antidepressant monotherapy." In other words, for many people, if you add LMF to antidepressants—the antidepressants work better!

For example, in two of the four studies, the addition of LMF to the antidepressant regimen more than doubled the number of people who responded to antidepressants—from 15 percent of patients to 32 percent. In another of the studies—a so-called "real-world" study (with the data used in the study collected from patient records and other real-world sources)—68 percent of patients responded to antidepressants only after LMF was added to the therapy.

The researchers point out that the therapy is particularly effective in people who are obese and have high levels of inflammatory biomarkers. And they contrast LMF to commonly used "adjunctive" medical treatments like atypical antipsychotic drugs, emphasizing that LMF does *not* cause the type of adverse side effects often caused by those drugs.[10]

"Sustained remission and recovery." In a study reported in the *Journal of Clinical Psychiatry*, sixty-eight treatment-resistant patients who had participated in a clinical trial on adding LMF to antidepressants were given the opportunity to participate in a yearlong study in which they could continue to take LMF. The success over the year was astounding:

- Of the sixty-eight people who participated, twenty-six (38 percent) achieved full recovery, with no recurrence of major depression.

- Of those sixty-eight, fifty-seven people entered the study as non-remitted—and thirty-five (61 percent) achieved remission.

Vitamin D Protects Your Brain

I discuss vitamin D and its importance for brain health—and relieving depression—in Chapter 5. A study published in 2024 shows just how powerful vitamin D is—particularly if you're taking an antidepressant.

The researchers looked at forty-six people with MDD, dividing them into two groups—one took vitamin D, and one took a placebo. After seven months, those with the highest increase in blood vitamin D had the most relief from depressive symptoms (and anxiety).

"More importantly," wrote the researchers in *Psychological Medicine*, brain scans showed that those *not* taking vitamin D had "disrupted integrity" in areas of the brain over those seven months, and less connectivity between parts of the brain.

The researchers' conclusion: "Vitamin D supplementation as an adjunctive [additional] therapy to antidepressants may not only contribute to improvement in clinical symptoms but also help preserve brain structural and functional connectivity in major depressive disorder patients."[11]

Protecting your brain from injury while taking antidepressants—one more compelling reason to make sure you optimize your blood levels of vitamin D with targeted nutritional supplementation.

This evidence demonstrates "sustained remission and sustained recovery" from adding 15 mg a day of LMF to the treatment regimen of people who don't adequately respond to an antidepressant, concluded the researchers from the Department of Psychiatry at Rush University in Chicago.[12]

If your antidepressant isn't working for you; if you're obese, with a body mass index of 30 or higher; if you have high levels of an inflammatory biomarker like C-reactive protein (CRP); or if you have markers for a genetic mutation of the methylenetetrahydrofolate reductase (MTHFR) gene, with controls the conversion of folate to LMF—you are *definitely* a candidate for augmentation with LMF.

And I'm far from the only one with this perspective. A study from researchers in the Department of Psychiatry at Harvard Medical School, published in the *Journal of Clinical Psychiatry*, came to the same conclusion, albeit stated in dense scientific terms:

"Biomarkers associated with inflammation or metabolism and genomic markers associated with L-methylfolate synthesis and metabolism may identify patients with SSRI-resistant depression who are responsive to adjunctive therapy with L-methylfolate."[13]

Magnesium

As you read in Chapter 7, magnesium plays a key role in the formation of neurotransmitters, particularly mood-regulating serotonin and pleasure-supplying dopamine. It also helps serotonin bind to neurons and transmit its messages. And low magnesium can interfere with glutamate receptors, causing damage to neurons from overstimulation.

Scientific research testifies to the power of magnesium to augment antidepressants:

Magnesium improves the effectiveness of SSRIs. In research published in December 2022, four university-based psychiatrists studied sixty people with MDD who were taking an SSRI, dividing them into two groups: one group received a daily dose of magnesium; the other group received a placebo. The researchers tested for depression levels at the beginning of the study, and after six weeks, using the Beck Depression Inventory. On average, those taking magnesium for six weeks had much lower scores than those taking the placebo, with improvements in symptoms like sadness, guilt, self-hate, irritability, insomnia, fatigue, and suicidality. Magnesium, wrote the researchers in the *Journal of Family Medicine and Primary Care*, "can be considered as a potential adjunct treatment option for MDD patients who are under SSRI treatment." In other words: if you're taking an SSRI, take magnesium, too.[14]

Eighty-eight percent achieve remission—with Prozac *and* magnesium. Researchers at the University of Warsaw in Poland looked at ninety-one people who had been hospitalized for MDD. Thirty-nine were given tricyclic antidepressants; thirty-five were given Prozac; and seventeen were given Prozac *and* magnesium. The best results? The seventeen patients taking the Prozac/magnesium combo, with fifteen patients achieving remission after eight weeks. These results were reported in the July 15, 2021, issue of the *Journal of Clinical Medicine*.[15]

And in a study published in the August 3, 2018, issue of *Nutrients*, the same team of researchers studied thirty-seven people with recurrent depression—giving them either: 1) Prozac; 2) Prozac and magnesium (120 mg daily of magnesium aspartate); or 3) Prozac and a placebo. "Treatment augmentation with magnesium," wrote the researchers, "increased the odds of effective treatment."[16]

As I pointed out in the section on magnesium in Chapter 7, one way that SSRIs may work is by increasing levels of magnesium in the brain. Why not support the medication with a magnesium supplement?

Probiotics

As you've read in Chapter 11—"Repairing the Gut-Brain Network"—increasing the friendly bacteria in the gut with a probiotic supplement can play a key role in regulating mood. And as an August 2023 study in *JAMA Psychiatry* revealed, a probiotic supplement can boost the power of antidepressants.

Thirty percent fewer depressive symptoms—with probiotics. The study was conducted by a team of researchers in England, at the prestigious King's College London and several other institutions. The researchers wanted to answer this question: "Are probiotics an acceptable, tolerable, and potentially efficacious adjunctive treatment for depression?" ("Adjunctive" here means adding the probiotics to antidepressant treatment.)

To find out, they studied forty-nine people with MDD who were taking an antidepressant but had an "incomplete response." They divided them into two groups: twenty-four people received a probiotic supplement with many different strains (types) of friendly bacteria; the other twenty-five received a placebo. Four and eight weeks into the study, the researchers tested the participants for depressive symptoms. The results:

The people taking the probiotics had a 30 percent greater improvement in depressive symptoms compared to the placebo group.

Lithium

"The First-Choice Treatment"

In Chapter 8, I discussed low-dose *nutritional* lithium orotate for depression, starting with 2 mg daily. Well, *pharmaceutical* lithium carbonate is used as an augmentation for people who do not respond to antidepressants.

An analysis of nine studies on augmenting antidepressants with lithium led the authors to conclude that "lithium augmentation is the first-choice treatment procedure for depressed patients who fail to respond to antidepressant [therapy]."[17]

Now, if antidepressants are working for you, I'm not recommending you go to your doctor and ask to be put on high-dose lithium carbonate. But I am suggesting that these studies show it could be a smart move to add low-dose nutritional lithium orotate to your augmentation regimen.

In my clinical experience, and in the experience of thousands of clinicians who I have trained in Functional Psychiatry, augmenting with 2 to 20 mg of lithium orotate can be very helpful.

Another measurement—the Inventory of Depressive Symptomatology—showed the probiotic group had 36 percent greater improvement. The probiotic group also had 21 percent greater improvements in anxiety symptoms.[18]

So, yes, the study proved that probiotics are a "potentially efficacious adjunctive treatment"—in other words, if you're taking an antidepressant, add a probiotic supplement to your regimen.

Additionally, only one of the twenty-four people taking the probiotics stopped taking them during the study, and no one had an adverse reaction to the supplement—answering the questions about whether probiotics are "acceptable" and "tolerable" with a big *yes*.

Symptoms reduced by 18 percent. A meta-analysis showed that adding probiotics to antidepressants provides an additional reduction of depressive symptoms of 18 percent. That study was published in the February 8, 2021, issue of the *Journal of Clinical Medicine*. The authors of the meta-analysis theorized that probiotics may work by boosting levels of brain-derived neurotropic factor (BDNF) and decreasing inflammation.[19] (I talk much more about the mechanism of action of probiotics in Chapter 11.)

Rhodiola Rosea

I talked about the herb *Rhodiola rosea* in Chapter 10. As I said there, it stops the breakdown of the neurotransmitters dopamine and norepinephrine, improving depressive symptoms. It can also boost the power of antidepressant medication.

Best results: Zoloft and *Rhodiola*. In a study conducted by Chinese psychiatrists at Fujian Traditional Chinese Medical University, 100 people with mild to moderate depression were divided into three groups. Each group received three pills per day:

- Group A—Zoloft, and two placebos

- Group B—Zoloft, and two *Rhodiola* capsules (600 mg daily)

- Group C—Zoloft, one *Rhodiola* capsule (300 mg daily), and one placebo

Group B had the biggest reduction in depressive symptoms. *Rhodiola* "shows antidepressive potency in patients with depressive disorder," concluded the researchers, in the March 15, 2020, issue of *Journal of Affective Disorders*.[20]

Polyphenols

In Chapter 10, I also discussed oligomeric proanthocyanidins (OPCs), plant compounds that balance and energize the brain in many ways, helping to relieve depression. The best way to get OPCs for augmentation of an antidepressant is through *extracts,* supplements that contain high levels of OPCs—specifically, grape seed extract, blueberry extract, green tea extract, and pine bark extract. One of the best studies on OPCs and antidepressants was conducted with pine bark extract— using the supplement to reverse sexual dysfunction triggered by an antidepressant.

Sexual dysfunction is a common side effect of antidepressants, with a study in the *Journal of Clinical Psychiatry*[21] showing that six out of ten people taking an antidepressant develop this problem. And 60 percent is a conservative figure. In one study, 93 percent of men and women taking Anafranil (clomipramine) suffered from either partial or total anorgasmia, the inability to have an orgasm.[22]

The types of sexual side effects caused by antidepressants include: less sexual desire (low libido); less sexual excitement (and even complete loss of sensation in the penis or vagina); diminished or delayed orgasm; erectile dysfunction; and painful ejaculation. Pine bark extract can counter those side effects.

After one month—fewer sexual side effects. In a study published in the March 1, 2019, issue of *Physiology International*, researchers in eastern Europe studied seventy-two people with depression who were taking Lexapro (escitalopram). They divided them into two groups: Thirty-seven took Lexapro *and* Pycnogenol, a pine bark extract; thirty-five continued to take Lexapro only. After one month of treatment, those who were taking Pycnogenol had much less sexual dysfunction. The researchers speculate the pine bark extract worked by improving circulation and reducing inflammation.[23]

Curcumin

In the chapter on OPCs, I also discussed curcumin, the active ingredient of the spice turmeric. It, too, can play a role in your augmentation protocol.

Less inflammation, less depression. Chinese scientists studied 108 men taking antidepressants, adding either curcumin (2,000 mg) or a placebo to their daily regimen. After six weeks, the men taking the curcumin had lower biomarkers of inflammation, increased levels of the BDNF (which energizes and protects neurons), and "significant antidepressant behavioral response." Curcumin, wrote the researchers in the *Journal of Clinical Psychopharmacology*, can "enhance the outcome of antidepressants treatment in major depressive disorder."[24]

Final thoughts

As you can see from this chapter, there are *many* natural, nondrug compounds that can improve the effectiveness and reduce the side effects of an antidepressant. If you're on an antidepressant but not satisfied with the results, I strongly urge you to share the information in this chapter with your physician and discuss an augmentation approach.

A few key points:

- If you are on an antidepressant, make sure your vitamin D level is checked and supplementation is optimized to achieve a level of 40 to 60.

- Make sure your vitamin B12 level is checked, and optimized to over 500.

After that testing and supplementation is completed, you could also add:

- Broad spectrum multivitamin-mineral supplement that includes zinc (no less than 15 mg)

- B complex supplement that includes LMF

- Magnesium glycinate (240 mg daily, 120 mg morning and 120 mg evening)

- Curcumin and OPCs, in the form of CurcumSorb Mind, two pills daily

CHAPTER 16

Understanding Antidepressant Deprescribing

> Forty million Americans take antidepressants—and twenty million are at risk for debilitating symptoms if they try to discontinue the drug. If you want to stop antidepressants, here's what you need to know.

Depression as a disease has been around since the birth of civilization, with the ancient Greeks describing it as *melancholia*, which they thought was caused by an excess of black bile—and which they treated with uplifting music and poetry, and with religious rituals and dream therapy. But as medicine has evolved over the millennia, so has the understanding of depression—and its treatment.

The First Antidepressants

The first antidepressants—monoamine oxidase inhibitors (MAOIs) and tricyclics—were marketed in the United States starting in the 1950s. The specific mechanism of action of these two classes of drugs wasn't understood when they were introduced. Now, it's understood that MAOIs work by inhibiting the activity of the enzyme *monoamine oxi-*

dase, which breaks down neurotransmitters like serotonin, dopamine, and norepinephrine. And tricyclics work by blocking the "reuptake" of serotonin and norepinephrine, allowing the neurons that release these neurotransmitters to reabsorb them, increasing their availability.

Neurotransmitters affect nearly *every* aspect of brain function and behavior. They directly regulate mood, memory, learning, sleep, the movement of muscles, and much more. Not surprisingly, early formulations of these drugs had numerous side effects, and high doses were toxic. As such, they were prescribed carefully: on a limited basis, and with strict regimens of monitoring.

The Neurotransmitter Hypothesis

Fast-forward a decade to the 1960s. Low neurotransmitter levels were hypothesized to be the *main cause* of depression. The core idea: Depression is caused by a lack of serotonin or other neurotransmitters. And since antidepressant medications were hypothesized to increase the availability of neurotransmitters in the brain, the medical industry assumed the drugs could and would *cure* depression.

The concept of depression as a disorder with a straightforward cause and cure in the brain's chemistry proved to be a highly marketable idea. (As research into depression continued and progressed, it became increasingly clear that the cause of the disorder was far more complex than a simple lack of a few brain chemicals. More about that in a moment.)

And pharmaceutical companies were more than willing to advertise their antidepressant medications as "cures" for neurotransmitter deficits.

The Prozac Revolution

Prozac was the first drug in a new category of antidepressant medications: selective serotonin reuptake inhibitors (SSRIs). Prozac entered the market in 1988 amid a wave of hype and promising results from clinical trials. Not only was it effective, said the drug's manufacturer, but it was also safe, with a range of potential applications that extended beyond the treatment of depression. In fact, it wasn't long before marketers were touting Prozac as a way to augment personality and performance.

"Are you too shy?" asked one advertisement. "Prozac can help."

"Do you need more ambition to reach that job promotion?" asked another. "Try Prozac to boost your motivation."

And this marketing worked. Big-time.

With the need for an effective therapeutic solution for depression as pressing as ever, and with the lines between a medicine and a personality modifier beginning to blur, Prozac quickly became a household name, a new "magic bullet" to cure not only depression but personal weaknesses, flaws, and shortcomings.

After all, if a single pill could banish the blues *and* give your personality a boost, why question anything about it?

Demand for Prozac and other antidepressant medications skyrocketed. Meanwhile, the long-term side effects and emerging withdrawal symptoms of Prozac were swept under the rug (if they were even noticed in the first place).

Profits over Health

By 1990, Prozac was the country's most prescribed antidepressant, with annual sales exceeding one billion dollars. But cracks began to emerge in Prozac's carefully crafted image.

After starting the drug, previously stable individuals reported uncontrollably violent thoughts, including self-directed suicidal violence. People appeared on talk shows, talking about the psychological horrors of being on Prozac, and describing themselves as "Prozac survivors." Many commentators noted—correctly—that antidepressants were being prescribed far too liberally, especially considering the fact that science still lacked a precise understanding of how the drugs worked, and of the biology of depression itself.

At the same time, psychiatrists began to hear from patients that stopping antidepressants produced withdrawal symptoms—symptoms that were often debilitating. And prolonged.

Specifically, patients who tried stopping Prozac and related antidepressants reported dizziness, lightheadedness, paresthesia (burning or tinging in the extremities), anxiety, gastrointestinal problems, poor coordination, headaches, "brain zaps," insomnia, irritability, tremors, and more.

Those symptoms were markedly similar to the withdrawal symptoms seen with stopping benzodiazepine medications like Valium.

Understanding Depression

Fast-forward once again, to the twenty-first century. Neurotransmitters—particularly serotonin—are still presumed to play key roles in the development of depressive disorders. But with decades of additional research—including brain imaging and genetic assay technology—we now know there are *many* causes of depression, and their interrelationship is very complex.

Those causes can be: genetic (DNA); epigenetic (modifications of DNA expression); metabolic (processes that convert nutrients and other compounds into energy); and biochemical (molecules that play essential roles in the body). External factors—from family dynamics to lifestyle—also can play a role in the development of depression.

Bottom line: Depression is much more than an imbalance of neurotransmitters. It has many genetic (inborn), psychological (stress/trauma), and environmental (external) factors, with the latter including the "environment" of your diet, your relationships, your work, where you live, etc.

You would think that with all of these advancements in the understanding of depression, we would have updated how we treat the disorder. But when it comes to depression, the gap between medical understanding and medical practice has *widened*. Substantially.

Depression is still treated in very much the same way it was treated fifty years ago: with medications thought to work by targeting neurotransmitter levels.

Unfortunately, there is still a lot of depression to treat.

Forty Million Prescriptions

More than twenty-one million American adults—about one in eight of us—suffer from a major depressive episode in any given year. During the years of the pandemic, that number more than tripled to seventy-two million American adults—about one in four of us.

How has mainstream psychiatry attempted to treat this epidemic of depression?

By prescribing more pills, of course.

In a recent year, forty million Americans filled a prescription for an antidepressant medication. Of those forty million, ten million have been on an antidepressant for a decade or longer.

And these numbers are climbing.

During the COVID-19 pandemic, more Americans than ever turned to antidepressants to banish the blues and calm their nerves. Prescriptions for antidepressants rose 19 percent between February and March 2020, when the pandemic started in the United States in full force.

In the middle of the biggest pandemic in a century, with people stressed, afraid, and worried about getting sick, more people than ever turned to doctors for help with depression. And the solution was usually an antidepressant—a drug that carries risks for severe withdrawal.

Bottom line: More Americans than ever will experience and struggle with antidepressant dependence and withdrawal. Perhaps you're one of them.

SSRI Antidepressants: The New Valium?

When scientific evidence shows that a popular psychoactive drug is in fact addictive, with withdrawal symptoms, the pharmaceutical industry and mainstream medicine respond in a predictable way—mainly, with denial, delay, and obfuscation, so they can eke every last dollar out of the drug. Case in point:

Valium (diazepam) was first released in the United States in 1963 as an improved version of older benzodiazepine formulations used to treat anxiety disorders, a problem that currently afflicts one in five American adults. More potent than its predecessor Librium, Valium quickly became a pharmaceutical bestseller, earning the rank of top-selling pharmaceutical in the United States from 1969 to 1982. At the height of its popularity in the mid-1970s, approximately 14 percent of Americans filled prescriptions for Valium, with more than two billion tablets sold yearly.

Throughout the 1970s, professional (and public) opinion was almost entirely in favor of Valium. Reports showed the drug might create dependency and addiction. But those reports were either ignored or dismissed.

For example, the chief of clinical pharmacology at Massachusetts General Hospital (the teaching hospital of Harvard Medical School) was quoted in a 1976 issue of *The New Yorker* as saying, "I have never seen a case of benzodiazepine dependence." And, he added, such addiction to Valium would be "an astonishingly unusual event."[1]

Given the addictive reality of the drug, there was *some* opposition to Valium and other benzodiazepines. In 1974, a *New York Times* article included quotes from physicians who questioned the prevailing wisdom that Valium represented an unfailingly safe and effective treatment for anxiety.[2] But most primary care physicians and psychiatrists continued to prescribe Valium without a second thought.

The tide of treatment began to shift in the early 1980s, as research started to generate data that became increasingly difficult for health professionals to ignore.

Multiple studies replicated this fundamental finding: Not only was benzodiazepine dependence and withdrawal real, but it was also occurring at *prescribed levels* of the drug.

I'm recounting this history of Valium because the dismissal of benzodiazepine dependency and withdrawal is strikingly similar to the current dismissal of dependency and withdrawal with SSRIs. In other words, professional opinion and practice about antidepressants has followed a trajectory nearly identical to that of Valium: 1) denial; 2) begrudging admission of the reality of dependency; 3) downplaying of its clinical relevance.

Valium and Antidepressants

The Same Set of Withdrawal Symptoms

Dependency on benzodiazepines like Valium, Ativan, and Xanax is a real phenomenon—and so is dependency on SSRIs (and the antidepressant drugs called selective norepinephrine reuptake inhibitors, or SNRIs). In fact, the symptoms of withdrawal from benzodiazepines and antidepressants are remarkably similar, as this list of symptoms common to both makes very clear:

Abdominal pain/cramping, agitation, aggressive behavior, amnesia, anorexia, anxiety, altered taste, ataxia (poor muscle control), blurred vision, chest pain, concentration problems, confusion, coordination problems, delirium, depersonalization and derealization (detachment from your thoughts and feelings), depression, diarrhea, dizziness, electric shock–like sensations, flu-like symptoms, flushing, headache, hyperesthesia (increased sensitivity to stimulation), insomnia, irritability, lethargy, lightheadedness, malaise, muscle spasms, myalgia (muscle pain), myoclonus (muscle twitching), nervousness, nightmares, numbness, pain, panic, paresthesia (burning or prickling sensations in the extremities), postural hypotension, restlessness, stiffness, sweating, tachycardia, tinnitus, tremor, vomiting, and weakness.

When they were first introduced, SSRIs were hailed as "wonder drugs," medications that represented a real answer to depression. They were marketed by the pharmaceutical industry—and subsequently viewed by the public—as a "quick-fix" solution for all types of depression, from mild to severe; a solution that came with little or no downside.

And this perspective has persisted, changing little since Prozac was first marketed in the late 1980s. At least it hasn't changed on the part of drug companies and most doctors. But this perspective is now increasingly at odds with scientific research.

A growing number of peer-reviewed analyses have confirmed this medical fact: Not only is antidepressant withdrawal a *real* phenomenon for some individuals, it is similar (and, for some, far worse) than the withdrawal symptoms associated with Valium and other benzodiazepines.

Why Isn't It Called "Antidepressant Withdrawal"?

After an abundance of research showing that antidepressant addiction and withdrawal was indeed a real risk, psychiatrists finally responded. And as I said in the previous section, the response was similar to that seen with Valium: *ignore* the facts; *deny* the facts; *downplay* the facts.

Even as thousands of individuals reported similar types of withdrawal symptoms as those seen with benzodiazepines, and it became evident that what they were experiencing was, in fact, withdrawal—psychiatrists didn't budge.

Instead, mainstream psychiatry made a concerted effort to "rebrand" the symptoms of antidepressant withdrawal as something relatively mild. To avoid the stigma (and potential loss of profits) from a negative term like "withdrawal," psychiatry simply established a new name.

The approved clinical term for withdrawal from SSRIs and SNRIs is: "antidepressant discontinuation syndrome," or ADS. The term "medication discontinuation syndrome" (MDS) is also used.

But this euphemism (a word meant to disguise a harsh reality, like calling a "prison" a "correctional facility") was not coined by psychiatrists.

The term was coined by a representative of the pharmaceutical giant Eli Lilly (the producer and marketer of Prozac), at a meeting of the Committee on Safety of Medicines in England, in 1998.[3] A summary of the meeting stated,

> The Committee was informed that Lilly . . . has expressed concern on the use of the term "withdrawal reaction" . . . due to the fact that "withdrawal" has a specific meaning and implies the drug is addictive. Lilly has suggested the use of the term "discontinuation reactions."[4]

In other words, presenting reliable, accurate information about addiction risks and withdrawal reactions—information that would fulfill basic requirements for informed consent—would potentially reduce the number of patients taking antidepressant medications.

(The term increasingly used by patients and doctors is "deprescribing," and it's the term I'll use for the rest of this chapter.)

The Scandal of Informed Consent (Too Often, There Isn't Any)

"Informed consent" means that patients are completely informed of both the benefits *and* risks of any proposed treatment.

Does characterizing antidepressant withdrawal as a "discontinuation syndrome" uphold the principle of informed consent?

The simple answer is: No.

In fact, a scientific review of physiologic, neurologic, and cognitive symptoms linked to SSRI antidepressant cessation concluded that referring to such symptoms as "discontinuation syndrome" is highly misleading!

Writing in *Psychotherapy and Psychosomatics*, the researchers stated that the appropriate terminology should be "withdrawal syndrome"—

since patients are clearly experiencing withdrawal from their medication when they try to stop it.[5]

Research indicates that up to 55 percent of patients experience significant withdrawal effects when they discontinue antidepressant medications. And 27 percent of patients report addiction (that is, the symptoms of withdrawal are so significant they *can't* stop the medication).[6]

These are significant numbers, with profound implications:

- **Forty million Americans** take an antidepressant medication.

- **Twenty million** are at risk of withdrawal upon discontinuation.

- **Ten million** struggle with antidepressant addiction.

The numbers speak for themselves: We are in a national crisis of antidepressant dependence and withdrawal.

What is the medical community doing about it? Nothing that works very well.

Current Approaches for Antidepressant Deprescribing

Given the number of antidepressants that are prescribed in the United States (and abroad), it would seem that developing clinical guidelines for deprescribing would be a matter of utmost importance to the medical establishment. But it's not.

The scientific literature on "best practices" for antidepressant deprescribing—that is, the best ways to help a patient withdraw from these drugs—is sparse.

Psychiatry continues to adhere to a largely symptom-based medication model of treating deprescribing. For example, if a patient develops diarrhea during deprescribing, they are prescribed an antidiarrheal medication; if the patient develops insomnia, they're prescribed a sleeping pill.

In essence, the psychiatric community remains steadfast in *minimiz-*

ing the importance of deprescribing—and fails to teach physicians how to help patients safely stop the addictive medications they prescribe.

But while psychiatry lacks official, comprehensive guidelines for deprescribing from antidepressants, several strategies actually do exist. However, these strategies are not formalized; they don't reflect a consensus; and they're based largely on clinical experiences and personal preferences of individual physicians. I have grouped these strategies into seven categories:

1. **Tapering based on symptoms.** "Tapering" is a slow discontinuation of a medication rather than stopping it "cold turkey." In this strategy, if symptoms from deprescribing are concerning, the doctor temporarily increases the medication dose, and then resumes the taper more slowly.

2. **Switch to another SSRI or SNRI antidepressant with a longer half-life.** The half-life of a drug is the time it takes for its concentration in the blood to be reduced by half. Drugs with longer half-lives may produce fewer acute deprescribing symptoms because their levels decrease more slowly over time. Switching to Prozac—which has a relatively long half-life—is often utilized as a deprescribing treatment strategy.

3. **Prescribe an atypical antipsychotic.** These drugs might help with symptoms. But they come with their own concerning side effects, like weight gain, increased cholesterol levels, and tardive dyskinesia (a potentially permanent movement disorder).

4. **Psychotherapy.** Psychoanalysis, cognitive behavioral therapy (CBT), and mindfulness-based stress reduction (MBSR) are often suggested as strategies to help deal with deprescribing symptoms.

5. **Exercise.** Physical exercise—which is helpful for depression itself—is often suggested as a way to decrease deprescribing symptoms.

6. **Phototherapy.** Phototherapy utilizes artificial light exposure as a way to synchronize a patient's circadian rhythms ("body clock"),

thereby normalizing the sleep/wake cycle and helping to balance mood.

7. **Give up.** Traditional psychiatry often recommends that a patient who finds it too difficult to come off their antidepressant medication *stay* on the medications indefinitely—even if the drug is no longer providing any therapeutic benefit.

My professional experience and opinion: I am struck by how *little* these suggestions offer the patient suffering from antidepressant withdrawal symptoms.

Although you can find all of the above-listed strategies discussed in scientific literature, almost none have been definitively verified by clinical trials. That is, the strategies are *ideas*, but they're not supported and confirmed by research. They're merely the ways mental health clinicians treat patients struggling with antidepressant discontinuation. (And it's important to note that psychiatrists are not taught or trained in these techniques—they're just using them, and hoping for the best.)

To get the clearest sense of the chaos and confusion around these deprescribing strategies, let's look at tapering, the process of slowly withdrawing the patient from medication.

Some reports suggest that the physician reduce a patient's antidepressant dosage by 25 percent each week—a taper of four weeks.

Others advise a longer taper, of between six and eight weeks.

Still other researchers assert that a four-month taper is best.

And some researchers claim the whole approach is useless: There is no advantage to be gained through tapering as compared to abrupt discontinuation.

Lacking consistent protocols for safely tapering patients off antidepressants, many psychiatrists simply give up.

If there is any consensus to be found in traditional psychiatry regarding antidepressant tapering, it is one of cynicism and defeat.

Or, as a study in the *American Journal of Psychiatry* put it: Since "depression is a chronic disorder, we recommend continued, potentially indefinite treatment to reduce the risk of relapse or recurrence."[7]

In other words, some of the leading researchers in this field claim the only method proven to mitigate symptoms from stopping antidepressants is not stop them!

To my mind, recommending permanent treatment with antidepressants as a way to prevent deprescribing symptoms is *unacceptable*. Nor is it necessary. Because there *is* a way to discontinue antidepressants with minimal (or no) side effects.

A Better, Safer Way to Stop Antidepressants

To effectively treat patients experiencing symptoms from antidepressant deprescribing, doctors *must* help patients manage their symptoms, as well as implement strategies to prevent depression relapse.

These are *exactly* the strategies you will find in this book.

In the next chapter, you will discover a safe, science-supported, patient-proven protocol for ending dependency on antidepressants. A protocol I've used successfully with hundreds of patients.

Hyperbolic Tapering— Conventional Psychiatry Gets More Individualized

I'm very happy to see a new approach to antidepressant deprescribing that mirrors the type of deprescribing I describe in this book: hyperbolic tapering, or tapering *very* slowly, making sure to avoid withdrawal symptoms as much as possible.

It's called *hyperbolic* because the tapering method is gradual rather than following a strict, linear reduction. (In geometry, a hyperbola is type of curve.) In hyperbolic tapering, the dose reductions become progressively smaller as the patient approaches zero dosage—and this patient-centered reduction always keeps the patient's comfort foremost.   *(continued)*

In a study published in *Therapeutic Advances in Psychopharmacology*, on May 9, 2023, Dutch researchers looked at nearly four thousand patients who were deprescribing. They found standard tapering produced more withdrawal symptoms than hyperbolic tapering. "Antidepressant tapering in clinic practice requires a *personalized process* [emphasis mine] of shared decision-making over the entire course of the tapering period," they wrote.[8] Agreed!

And more professionals *are* agreeing. An article in the September 19, 2023, issue of the *Pharmaceutical Journal* (a U.K. publication) discussed the facts of antidepressant withdrawal ("It is now recognized that withdrawal effects from antidepressants are more common, and can be more severe and long-lasting."), and noted that "newly updated National Institute of Health and Care Excellence and Royal College of Psychiatrists guidelines recommend hyperbolic/proportional tapering."[9] (Let's hope the U.S. health care system follows suit.)

A shortcoming of the hyperbolic approach, however, is that it does *not* use targeted nutritional supplementation to support the deprescribing process. Patient-centered, slow tapering *and* nutritional support is the best method.

That protocol is largely based on the nutritional strategies you read about in Part II of this book. Here's why the protocol works.

Antidepressant medications modulate levels of specific neurotransmitters, particularly serotonin, the "feel-good" neurotransmitter.

In response, the brain requires a higher level of serotonin to sustain what has become the new biochemical "normal."

When the antidepressant medication is discontinued, the brain's demand for higher levels of serotonin more often than not leads to a wide range of physical and psychological effects. (Remember, 55 percent of people who try to stop their antidepressant experience these symptoms.)

Many of the nondrug treatments I recommend for reducing and

eliminating antidepressant deprescribing symptoms affect serotonin synthesis—and optimizing serotonin levels prevents, relieves, or reverses the symptoms of withdrawal (while also providing significant mental health benefits).

These natural treatments include:

- free amino acids (Chapter 4);

- vitamin D (Chapter 5);

- vitamin B12, folate, and other B vitamins (Chapter 6);

- zinc, magnesium, and other trace minerals (Chapter 7);

- essential fatty acids (EFAs; Chapter 9); and

- polyphenols found in colorful plants like blueberries and red grapes (Chapter 10).

If you and your doctor decide not to discontinue antidepressants, Chapter 15 offers a nutritional program to improve pharmaceutical performance, and to prevent side effects from antidepressants, like weight gain and sexual dysfunction.

My Essential Message

If you are on antidepressants and want to get off these drugs, my essential and optimistic message to you is this:

Yes, there *is* a path forward.

Yes, there *are* effective techniques to help you safely stop taking antidepressant medications.

The first step is identifying the underlying nutritional deficiencies with *testing*.

The second step is supporting the production of serotonin and other neurotransmitters (and other aspects of brain neurochemistry) with *treatment*, emphasizing natural therapies.

And the next chapter describes the way to take those steps—because it provides all the principles and practical answers you need to deal with antidepressant deprescribing and minimize symptoms of withdrawal.

One final note: I have written a book for health professionals that presents a comprehensive review of antidepressant withdrawal: *Functional Medicine for Antidepressant Withdrawal: An Integrative and Functional Medicine Approach to the Treatment and Prevention of Antidepressant Withdrawal.* If your health professional wants an in-depth and practical presentation on this topic, please let them know about the book, which is available at www.jamesgreenblattmd.com.

CHAPTER 17

The Antidepressant Deprescribing Plan

> A safe and patient-proven protocol for ending your dependency on antidepressants.

Selective serotonin reuptake inhibitors (SSRIs) and selective serotonin-norepinephrine reuptake inhibitors (SNRIs) are the most commonly prescribed antidepressant, in America and around the world.

Are these medications effective?

Well, that's a debate that has raged for decades. I don't expect it to be resolved anytime soon. In my clinical experience, SSRIs and SNRIs work wonderfully well for some people, and not so well for others.

But what is not debatable is that SSRIs and SNRIs have a profound effect on the way your brain functions. As their name says, they block the "reuptake" of serotonin into the neuron that released it. That action makes more serotonin available in the synaptic gap—the space between neurons. As a result, serotonin can bind to the serotonin receptors on the surface of neurons for longer periods of time, improving neuron-to-neuron signaling along the pathways that regulate mood.

This physiological process tells the body that there's more serotonin on board. As a result, the body actually *decreases* the production of serotonin.

Which means that when you stop taking the SSRI/SNRI, your body can go into a kind of serotonin shock from low levels of serotonin, with headaches, brain zaps (an electric shock-like or tinging sensation that occurs in the brain or throughout the body), irritability, insomnia, intense agitation, and even suicidality.

But here's the thing. Not everybody has these withdrawal symptoms!

In fact, if you take a group of people of the same age, who have been taking an SSRI for the same amount of time—about half will have withdrawal symptoms, and about half won't.

Well, what I've discovered through laboratory testing is that the people with the worst withdrawal symptoms have the most significant nutritional deficiencies!

That's why the core of the Antidepressant Deprescribing Plan is working with your doctor to find those nutritional deficiencies and fix them—*before* your doctor tapers the antidepressant. By doing that, you and your doctor dramatically decrease the likelihood of significant withdrawal symptoms.

That's because several nutrients—like zinc, vitamin D, folate, B6, and B12—are essential cofactors in the creation of serotonin. If you're deficient in one of those nutrients, or you're genetically programmed with a need for higher levels of the nutrient, or your diet is deficient in that nutrient—when your doctor begins to taper the SSRI/SNRI, and your body tries to start producing more serotonin, it's not going to happen, because you're lacking the raw materials for serotonin manufacture. And guess what? You're going to have withdrawal symptoms.

Bottom line: To safely deprescribe from SSRIs/SNRIs, you and your doctor need to *test* for the levels of these nutrients, use targeted nutritional supplementation to correct low levels, and only then can your doctor taper you off your SSRI/SNRI.

The Two Key Principles of the Plan

As I've just explained, finding and fixing nutritional deficiencies *before* tapering off an antidepressant is the essence of the Antidepressant Deprescribing Plan. These two steps are a must:

1) **Test** for the nutritional deficiencies or imbalances that contribute to deprescribing side effects.

    These deficiencies and imbalances are discussed at length in Part II. They include:
    - amino acids;
    - vitamin D;
    - B vitamins (B12, folate, pyridoxine);
    - minerals (zinc, magnesium, lithium); and
    - essential fatty acids.

2) **Treat** nutritional deficiencies and imbalances, establishing a baseline of biochemical health.

For Antidepressant Deprescribing, the Doctor *Must* Be In

In Part II of this book, you discovered the nutrients that balance brain chemistry—and that can prevent or treat depression. Many of the nutritional supplements I presented in Part II—like free-form amino acids, zinc, and magnesium—can be taken on your own without testing or monitoring. Well, those very same nutrients are the practical basis of the Antidepressant Deprescribing Plan: These nutrients normalize levels of serotonin, which decreases depressive symptoms; and *then* you can safely withdraw from the drug. But although the same nutrients are involved, it is *not* safe or effective to withdraw from antidepressants on your own. There are simply too many challenges and difficulties, like insomnia, anxiety, worsening depression, and physical symptoms. To deal with those difficulties, you need therapeutic support and a helping hand. Plus, you're dealing not only with self-care but with medical care—your doctor's area of expertise. Bottom line: To monitor and minimize the possible discomforts of deprescribing, and to ensure safety and success, you *must* work with your doctor.

In a moment, I'll provide all the details of the plan itself: a nutrient-by-nutrient review of the tests you need; the meaning of the results; and dosages to correct deficiencies and imbalances.

But first, I'd like to discuss the factors in the doctor-patient relationship that increase the likelihood of successful withdrawal.

Maximizing the Doctor-Patient Relationship for Successful Withdrawal

The path to recovery during antidepressant deprescribing can be full of challenges and difficulties. That's why it's important for you and your doctor to go on this journey *together*. And to do that successfully, there are several principles it is best for both you and your doctor to follow.

Establish a therapeutic alliance. You and your doctor should establish what I call a "therapeutic alliance"—an equal partnership, based on trust, with a nonjudgmental, expectation-free approach. In other words, your doctor shouldn't have a fixed idea of what antidepressant deprescribing looks like—and expect your process and the results to mirror that idea. Rather, your doctor should deprescribe with and for *you*, recognizing your individualized needs and responses. This type of mutuality is the foundation of good medicine—and the indispensable first step for an effective deprescribing plan.

Make sure your doctor understands your motivations to discontinue antidepressants. Your doctor should do their best to understand *your* motivations for wanting to stop taking antidepressant medications so they can be maximally involved in and supportive of your progress.

Perhaps you feel the drug is no longer beneficial—you're on antidepressants, but you're still depressed. Maybe you've heard antidepressants harm the brain. Maybe your family members or friends have been advising you to stop, and you've decided to listen to their advice. Understanding your rationale and motivations allows the doctor to work *with* you, to achieve your goals.

Test for and correct nutritional deficiencies *before* discontinuation. Before starting a taper of antidepressants, you should be free of depressive symptoms for a *minimum* of four to six months. (Often, longer is better.) In practical terms, that means your doctor should: 1) *test* you for nutritional deficiencies; and then 2) *treat* you for nutritional deficiencies. Antidepressant taper should start only *after* the deficiencies are corrected. This gives you the strongest possible foundation for antidepressant deprescribing *without* symptoms.

If you have a history of longstanding chronic depression, or you've had difficult antidepressant deprescribing experiences in the past, then you should be free of depressive symptoms for *at least six months to one year* before you start the antidepressant taper.

You need to collaborate with your doctor. When antidepressant medications are tapered, the doctor is a necessary part of the process, but the *patient* should be in the driver's seat—taking charge of his or her healing journey, with the doctor's advice and consent. The only exception to this rule is when the patient wants to taper too quickly—for best results, always go slow!

And remember, protocols that call for decreasing medications by a certain amount, per a fixed time frame—such as reducing the dose by 25 percent every two weeks—miss the point.

Every patient is unique. How *your* brain (and the rest of your body) reacts to decreasing your antidepressant dose will be unique. Tapering medication *slowly*, based on your needs and experiences, allows for a more personalized (and therefore more effective) approach.

Consider a compounding pharmacy. Unfortunately, most antidepressant medications do not come in forms that are conducive to slow tapering. I don't recommend "counting beads," the tiny particles found inside the capsules of some antidepressant medications. A reputable compounding pharmacy—a specialized pharmacy that creates customized medications from scratch for individual patients—can create custom dosing, making things easier for you and the doctor during the tapering process.

Monitor symptoms. If the taper is proceeding as it should, whenever you decrease a dose you should experience only *mild* symptoms, and only for a *few* days. Anxiety and insomnia are the most common symptoms of deprescribing. But again, if the taper is done correctly, these symptoms should always be mild and brief.

How to Find a Compounding Pharmacy near You

There are several organizations you can contact to find a compounding pharmacy and pharmacist:

International Academy of Compounding Pharmacists (IACP). This association represents compounding pharmacists, and offers a searchable directory of its members on their website. To find a compounding pharmacy near you, use the "Find a Compounder" feature on the home page of their website, www.iacprx.org.

Professional Compounding Centers of America (PCAA). This organization is a leading provider of compounding training and support for pharmacists. They have a membership directory on their website that allows you to search for compounding pharmacies that are part of their network. Go to www.pccarx.com, and click on the "Find a Compounder" link at the bottom of the page.

National Community Pharmacists Association (NCPA). This association represents independent community pharmacies. Their website has a directory that includes compounding pharmacies. Go to www.ncpanet.org, click the "Pharmacy Locator" link at the top of the page, and under "Find Your Local Pharmacy" choose the "Compounding" option in the drop-down menu.

Brain zaps—an electric shock–like or tingling sensation that occurs in the brain (or throughout the body)—are a frequent antidepressant deprescribing symptom. On an appropriate taper, brain zaps shouldn't happen. If you experience this symptom—or other severe symptoms, like dizziness, balance problems, or flu-like symptoms—you and your doctor should restore the previous dose. Your doctor should also retest you for nutritional deficiencies, because it's very likely a factor was missed that is now contributing to your side effects, and you need additional nutritional support. Your nutrient levels should return to normal *before* you reinitiate the taper.

Benefit from a maintenance dose. You and your doctor may find that you do better long-term *on* medication. If you're on a reduced dose and continue to struggle with further decreases—consider the reduced dose a success! There are some individuals that benefit from longer-term maintenance medication. (Remember, a nonjudgmental, expectation-free attitude is the very foundation of this process.) And you can use an antidepressant *and* nutritional supplements to boost the effectiveness and minimize the side effects of the maintenance dose, as described in Chapter 15.

Three other areas of importance for you and your doctor to keep in mind:

Withdrawal and relapse. There's a big difference between *withdrawal* and *relapse*.

Withdrawal symptoms of antidepressants, experienced during a safely and carefully implemented tapering process, are *short-lived*.

Relapse of depression (if it occurs) is the return of full-blown depressive symptoms, typically experienced one to three months after drug discontinuation. Your doctor should treat a relapse the same way as they treat any new case of depression.

Multiple medications. If you're on several psychoactive medications that you would like to taper, you should taper only one medication at a time—using the same principles of the doctor-patient relationship that I have discussed here.

PTSD. For patients with PTSD, tapering is often more complicated. Approach the process with caution, establishing biochemical balance first, and tapering very slowly.

And now it's time for you and your doctor to learn the details of the Antidepressant Deprescribing Plan. I have tested and proven this approach with thousands of my patients, and it has now been used by many other health providers in the United States and around the world. For the many patients who have been struggling and suffering from painful antidepressant deprescribing symptoms, this plan is the answer.

You no longer need to suffer from the limitations and inadequacies of conventional "one-size-fits-all" approaches to antidepressant discontinuation.

Resolving your depressive symptoms *is* possible.

Successful tapering with reduced side effects *is* possible.

Lasting recovery from depression without taking an antidepressant *is* possible.

And if you're ready, *now* is the time to begin.

I'm going to walk you and your doctor through this plan in the same order I introduced the nutrients in Part II. But since those nutrients are discussed so extensively in Part II, I'm not going to give you extensive background info about them; I'm going to cut right to the chase, concentrating mainly on the *tests* you need to *find* a deficiency, and the *treatments* you need to *fix* a deficiency. First test, then treat; find and fix—these are the essences of the Antidepressant Deprescribing Plan.

Amino Acids

Testing: Amino acids

Blood (plasma) and urine amino acid tests are available, and your doctor can use them to evaluate your amino acid status. My preference is testing blood/plasma levels.

However, even in patients *without* documented amino acid deficiency, or patients for whom testing is unavailable, I *still* recommend supplementation with free-form amino acids—because this supplement is remarkably effective at reducing depression and preventing deprescribing symptoms.

Supplementation: Free-form amino acids

I consider supplementing with free-form amino acids—amino acids that are not bound together as protein—to be *the* key component in the Antidepressant Deprescribing Plan. In fact, I *always* administer a free-form amino acid supplement, regardless of testing.

Free-form amino acids provide a readily available supply of *all* the necessary building blocks for neurotransmitters, enzymes, and amino acid–based hormones throughout the body. Eliminating amino acid deficiencies through supplementation often improves mood, focus, and energy levels.

If your diet is poor, or you have a gastrointestinal disorder that impairs normal digestion, free-form amino acids may be of exceptional importance and value. Providing amino acids in free form dramatically simplifies their digestion, absorption, and utilization.

Dose: 4 to 8 grams (g) per day.

Timing: 2 to 4 g, twice daily, on an empty stomach, before meals.

> **Important:** Twice per day intake is very important, because amino acids remain available within the body for only four to five hours.

Form: capsules or powder.

> You can mix powder-based, free-form amino acids in water or juice.

> **Important:** Don't mix your supplement in protein-rich liquids like yogurt or milk, which will compromise absorption. Likewise, don't take a capsule with milk.

> **Good news:** Free-form amino acids usually work quickly, with many patients noting positive changes in just a few weeks: elevated mood, improved mental clarity, better ability to cope with stress, and enhanced sleep.

Vitamin D

Testing

Your doctor should test for the "storage form" of the vitamin: 25-hydroxy vitamin D. The active form—1,25-hydroxy vitamin D—is not as accurate a marker for whether or not you have a deficiency or a low level of vitamin D.

Finally Hopeful Success Story

PATIENT: Pam

TREATMENT FOR: Antidepressant deprescribing

Pam was a sixty-two-year-old physician with a history of depression. She had been taking Zoloft (sertraline) for twenty years, at a dose of 200 mg daily, and her depression was under control. But she wanted to see if life was possible without the drug.

Pam had consulted with several psychiatrists and naturopathic doctors during the two years before she saw me—and was feeling quite discouraged in her quest to deprescribe. Anytime she tried to reduce her dosage—even by small amounts—she would experience unbearable withdrawal symptoms, like insomnia, irritability, agitation, severe nausea, and brain zaps.

In my history and clinical examination, I found that Pam was healthy, didn't take any other medications, and ate a good diet, rich in protein and good fats. She exercised regularly, including a mix of brisk walking, yoga, and strength training with a personal trainer. She also meditated daily. But even with all these supportive lifestyle practices in place, she would "spiral" (her word) every time she attempted to lower her dose of medication.

As with all my patients, I ordered a range of laboratory testing. The tests revealed that Pam was low in many amino acids and minerals, in spite of her good diet. This is a frequent finding in older adults, whose absorption of nutrients declines with age.

I recommended the following protocol for Pam:

Digestive enzymes with betaine hydrochloric acid (HC1), two capsules with each meal. This supplement supplied the necessary digestive support to help Pam absorb amino acids, nutrients that are a must for the creation of neurotransmitters. And adequate levels of neurotransmitters are a must for any deprescribing plan.

Free-form amino acid powder, 1 scoop, twice daily, between meals. Pam was low in amino acids, a foundation of brain health.

Trace mineral supplement, one capsule daily. Pam was low in minerals, many of which are also key in neurotransmitter formation.

B complex, one capsule daily. The extra brain- and nerve-balancing B vitamins were a kind of insurance policy against side effects from deprescription like insomnia, anxiety, irritability, agitation, and brain zaps.

Magnesium glycinate, 120 milligrams (mg), two times daily. Ditto for the magnesium. I chose the glycinate form because of its high absorbability, its gentleness on the digestive tract, and because both magnesium and glycine (an amino acid) can help with anxiety and insomnia.

I saw Pam a month later. She said she had more energy, less bloating after meals, and better sleep. At that point, we decreased her dose of Zoloft by 12.5 mg, and I asked her to see me in two weeks, to review her progress.

When I saw her again, Pam was excited to tell me that she had tolerated the dose reduction without significant adverse side effects—no brain zaps, no nausea, no insomnia. "I felt a little more irritable," she said. "But this dosage reduction has been so much better than any of the others. I can *function*."

She was delighted with her progress, and hoped she could continue to slowly decrease her dose of Zoloft.

Over the months, Pam continued her protocol, and successfully managed to decrease her Zoloft to 50 mg, without side effects. But at 50 mg, she began to experience high levels of irritability and anxiety. I did another round of testing.

Her amino acids levels had normalized. And Trace Mineral Hair Analysis showed that levels of most minerals had improved. But she was low in lithium, a mineral I consider key to brain health. We continued her protocol, adding 1 mg of lithium orotate. We also added the supplement SeroPlus from Pure Encapsulations, which boosts serotonin levels, using two capsules, twice daily, between meals.

With the addition of these supplements, Pam was able to continue her deprescription process. As of today, the supplements are still working, she no longer takes the antidepressants—and she still feels great.   *(continued)*

This Finally Hopeful Success Story is real-world evidence that you *can* slowly deprescribe from antidepressants, *without* significant side effects, *if* you use the Antidepressant Deprescribing Plan—the essence of which is: *first test, then treat.*

Results: A severe deficiency is a level under 20 nanograms per milliliter (ng/mL). Insufficiency is 20 to 30. Low-normal is 30 to 40. Optimal is 40 to 60.

If testing shows you should supplement with vitamin D—and almost everyone needs supplementation to restore optimal levels—your doctor should test you again three months after supplementation begins to ensure your dosage was adequate to optimize levels. After you have achieved optimal levels, you should be tested twice per year to confirm that levels are still in the optimal range. Increase your dosage if one of the biyearly tests shows that levels have fallen below optimal.

Important: Testing *before* supplementation is a must, because some people (but not many) maintain optimal vitamin D levels through dietary intake and sun exposure. If your levels are already optimal, and you begin taking vitamin D without testing, you could get too much of the vitamin.

Supplementation

Dose: 2,000 to 10,000 international units (IU) daily, based on testing.

Important: A common misconception about vitamin D is that once levels have been restored after a few months of treatment, you can discontinue supplementation. While abrupt discontinuation is unlikely to alter blood levels right away, it's likely you'll be deficient again within six months to a year of stopping vitamin D. The best strategy: daily adequate dosing, to proactively and consistently keep vitamin D levels in a healthy range. In patients with depression who have achieved optimum levels of blood vitamin D, I recommend 1,000 to 2,000 IU daily.

Timing: Take vitamin D once per day, with a meal that contains some fat, which maximizes absorption.

Form: Vitamin D comes in many forms, like pills, liquid, and gummies. Choose any form you like.

Vitamin B12

In Chapter 6, I wrote that confusion about vitamin B12 testing and supplementation is "one of the greatest tragedies in modern medicine"— because detecting and correcting low levels of B12 can do so much good. Restoring normal levels of vitamin B12 can defeat depression *and* restore energy *and* clear up brain fog *and* reduce the risk of cognitive decline (and much more). But low levels are routinely overlooked by conventional doctors.

I also wrote extensively about the *correct* process of vitamin B12 testing and supplementation: how to read results, and how to respond to them. For complete information, please read/review the B12 section in Chapter 6. Here, I'll cover the basics:

Testing

There are three tests that can show if you have low levels of vitamin B12:

Serum B12. Low (< 150 nanograms per liter, or ng/L) and even low-normal (< 500 ng/L) indicates a potential deficiency or need for supplementation.

Important: Normal levels (> 500 ng/L) do *not* rule out a need for supplementation.

Homocysteine: High (> 12 micromoles per liter, or µmol/L) can indicate deficiency of B12 (or folate).

Methylmalonic acid (MMA): High levels (> 245 nanomoles per liter, or nmol/L) can indicate deficiency or an increased need for B12.

But remember what I said in the chapter on B vitamins: normal values on any or all of these tests do not rule out a need for vitamin B12.

Supplementation

Dose and timing, intramuscular injections (IM): intramuscular B12, as hydroxocobalamin or methylcobalamin, 1,000 micrograms (µg) IM, three times per week.

Important: Injections work faster than oral supplementation to restore optimum B12 levels. Hydroxocobalamin is the precursor to active forms of vitamin B12 and is often used for injections. Methylcobalamin is the active form of B12 used by the tissues of the body and is often used for oral supplementation.

Also: It isn't unusual for blood B12 levels to become dramatically elevated after injections or supplementation. This is normal, and not a reason to discontinue treatment.

Dose and timing, oral supplementation: oral B12, as methylcobalamin, hydroxocobalamin, or adenosylcobalamin. 1,000 to 5,000 µg. *For example:* 2,000 µg, two times per day.

Form: sublingual. I recommend the product PureMelt B12 Folate, from Pure Encapsulations.

Important: When correcting B12 deficiency, B12 injections work more quickly, but sublingual B12 also works well.

Folate (Vitamin B9)

As I explain in Chapter 6, folic acid has historically been the main form of folate available for supplementation. Unfortunately, folic acid requires enzymatic transformation to the more active folates—a process that can be significantly impacted by methylenetetrahydrofolate reductase (MTHFR) gene variants, which are very common (up to 50 percent of the population). To prevent problems and maximize therapeutic benefits, supplementing with active folates is preferred.

Testing

Homocysteine: High levels (> 12 μmol/L) can indicate deficiency of folate (or vitamin B12).

MTHFR genetic testing for C677T and A1298C variants: Homozygous C677T (TT) and A1298C (CC) have increased requirements for L-methylfolate (LMF). Heterozygous C677T (CT) and A1298C (AC) often benefit from LMF supplementation as well.

Supplementation

Dose: 3 mg. If there is no improvement after one month, increase the dose to 5 to 10 mg.

Note: Occasionally, high doses of folate can cause agitation. To avoid this uncommon side effect, use the "start-low-and-go-slow" model. Begin with the low dose indicated here, and increase as indicated.

Form: L-methylfolate (LMF).

Important: Several classes of drugs interfere with folate metabolism, including birth control pills, antiseizure medications, antacids, and certain antibiotics (particularly sulfonamides like sulfamethoxazole and trimethoprim-sulfamethoxazole). Alcohol and tobacco also block folate. If possible, avoid them if you're attempting to restore folate levels.

Also: Any regimen of supplemental folate should include supplemental vitamin B12—because folate can mask a B12 deficiency, which can cause long-term nerve damage. As I said a moment ago, I recommend a B12/folate supplement: PureMelt B12 Folate, from Pure Encapsulations.

Pyridoxine (Vitamin B6)

Testing

Kryptopyrrole testing. As I discussed in Chapter 6, some individuals have high levels of kryptopyrroles, which bind with vitamin B6 and zinc, forcing these nutrients out of the body. In my clinical experience, patients with higher levels struggle with more intense symptoms during antidepressant deprescribing.

Testing for kryptopyrroles involves a random urine collection (i.e., not first thing in the morning), with patients off all supplements for twelve to twenty-four hours before the test. (Antibiotics can also interfere with the test.) Kryptopyrroles are somewhat unstable, degrading with light exposure; urine samples need to be handled properly to ensure accurate results.

Normal is 0–10 micrograms per deciliter (mcg/dL). Borderline is 11–15 mcg/dL. Elevated is above 15 mcg/dL.

Supplementation

If you have elevated levels of kryptopyrroles, you should take B6 and zinc.

Vitamin B6 dose: 50 to 100 mg per day.

Form: A fifty-fifty combination of pyridoxine and pyridoxal-5-phosphate (P5P, the active form of pyridoxine).

Important: After starting supplementation, I follow patients over the next month, watching for symptom improvement. In some cases, I may retest to determine how kryptopyrrole levels have responded to supplementation. If they are still high and symptoms still problematic, the dosage is increased to 100 mg of vitamin B6, two times per day.

Also: High levels of B6 have been linked to neuropathy. In general, supplementing with vitamin B6 up to 100 mg daily is considered safe (rarely, a patient develops neuropathy at daily doses below 200 mg). If caught early, vitamin B6 neuropathy can be reversed. If you start taking B6 and develop neuropathy—symptoms like tingling, numbness, and burning pain are common—stop taking B6.

Zinc dose: 60 mg per day.

Timing: 30 mg twice per day, with food.

Form: Zinc picolinate.

Important: Don't take zinc on an empty stomach; it can cause digestive upset.

Also: Long-term intake of zinc should not be above 30 mg per day to prevent copper deficiency, which can damage nerves and compromise the immune system.

Zinc

As I discussed in Chapter 7—if you're depressed, it's *very* likely you are low in zinc. In fact, one group of scientists concluded that zinc is so entwined with depression, the mineral could be considered a "biomarker of major depressive disorder." But testing for zinc levels is problematic: there is no standardized test to detect deficiency. All of which leads to the following strategies for testing and supplementation:

Testing

The most commonly used laboratory tests are serum zinc, the zinc-dependent enzymes alkaline phosphatase test, and the zinc-dependent white blood cell count. However, neither are definitive. Consider the Trace Mineral Hair Analysis, a hair test that measures zinc (among many other minerals). You could also use the Zinc Taste Test, discussed in Chapter 3.

Dosing

If you're depressed, it's likely you need more zinc.

> **Dose for those with depressive symptoms:** 60 mg per day.

> **Form:** Zinc picolinate.

> **Timing:** 30 mg, two times daily, with meals.

> **Dose for those in remission:** 30 mg per day.

> **Timing:** 15 mg, two times daily, with meals.

> **Important:** The cautions for zinc were covered in the section on B6.

Magnesium

Magnesium deficiency is *the* most common nutritional deficiency that I encounter in my clinical practice. But serum (blood) magnesium testing is *not* effective for identifying deficiencies—because 99 percent of magnesium is found in the bones, muscles, heart, and liver, with only 1 percent in the blood.

Testing

Trace Mineral Hair Analysis provides a simple, affordable, and useful tool for identifying magnesium deficiency.

> **Important:** There are also several clinical indicators of magnesium deficiency, including anxiety, insomnia, constipation, and health conditions that involve muscle spasms (asthma, muscle cramps, migraines, eye twitching, etc.).

Supplementation

Even without testing, I recommend a magnesium supplement for *every* patient with depression—because deficiency is so prevalent; and because magnesium is so safe and effective.

Dose: 240 mg, twice per day.

Form: Magnesium glycinate or magnesium citrate.

> **Important:** There are many different forms of supplemental magnesium, like magnesium glycinate, magnesium threonate, magnesium oxide, magnesium citrate, and magnesium gluconate. In my clinical experience, all of them are equally effective, with one exception: magnesium oxide, which is poorly absorbed.
>
> However, some people *may* respond better to one form of magnesium versus another, so it may be worthwhile to switch forms every couple of months and see if you derive more benefit from the new form.

Caution: The main side effect from taking magnesium is loose stools. This laxative effect is most common with magnesium oxide, another reason not to use it. If you develop loose stools, split or decrease the dose. Or switch to a slowly absorbed, long-acting form of magnesium.

Also: Some health experts recommend magnesium L-threonate as the best form of magnesium for the brain. That's because a few studies show brain-based benefits, like healthier brain cells and protection against age-related mental decline. There's nothing wrong with magnesium L-threonate, but it is more expensive than other forms. If you take magnesium threonate, the dose is 1,000 mg (which delivers 72 mg of elemental magnesium), twice per day.

Low-Dose Nutritional Lithium

I prescribe low-dose nutritional lithium to stabilize mood, to help with addictions, and to slow or stop memory loss in seniors. I also use it to help with depression—and the suicidality that is the most ominous symptom of depression.

Testing

While not necessary, Trace Mineral Hair Analysis is one of the simplest and most effective tests to assess lithium levels. Most people can benefit from low-dose lithium supplementation—although those with documented low hair levels have an even stronger need for the mineral.

Supplementation

As I just mentioned, I think that most individuals—depressed or healthy—can benefit from low-dose lithium supplementation.

But you're particularly likely to benefit from lithium if you have: irritability, anxiety, mood swings, compulsive behavior, or a history of self-injury; a previous or current psychiatric diagnosis, especially of depression, bipolar disorder, or borderline personality disorder, or a family history of those problems; or past or current substance abuse.

Dose: 2 to 10 mg per day.

Form: Lithium orotate.

Important: High-dose pharmaceutical lithium carbonate can cause serious side effects, including kidney disease, thyroid problems, and nerve damage. In contrast, low-dose nutritional lithium is very safe. It's been marketed and utilized worldwide for decades, and I've used it in thousands of patients without harmful side effects. However, there is not enough evidence to say that low-dose nutritional lithium is safe for pregnant women or women trying to conceive.

Essential Fatty Acids (EFAs)

EFAs are the building blocks of fat. They're also the building blocks of your brain, which is 60 percent fat by dry weight (meaning, if you drained all the water from the brain, the remaining material would be 60 percent fat).

Two of the most important EFAs are the omega-3s eicosapentaenoic acid (EPA) and docosahexaenoic acid (DHA), found mainly in fish oil. And deficiency of omega-3s is common. Our hunter-gatherer ancestors ate a diet with a ratio of about two to one omega-6s to omega-3s. Today, we eat a diet with the ruinous ratio of fifteen to one. (Omega-6s are found mostly in vegetable oils, mass-produced meats, and other processed foods.)

Testing

A common test for EFAs is called the Fatty Acid Profile. The most important result is the omega-6 to omega-3 ratio, which should be two to one.

But since deficiencies of omega-3 are so common, I think taking at least 3 g of omega-3 per day for three months *without* testing is safe. After three months of supplementation, take the test. If your ratio of omega-6s to omega-3s is not two to one, increase your dose of omega-3s.

Supplementation

The American Psychiatric Association recommends that people with mood disorders like depression supplement their diet with 1 or more g of a fish oil supplement, which supplies omega-3s. I recommend a somewhat higher level.

Dose: 3 g of fish oil per day.

Form: EPA to DHA ratio of three to one.

> **Caution:** The ocean is polluted, with toxins that accumulate in fish. Make sure your fish oil (or krill oil, or algae) omega-3 sup-

plement is from a company that adheres to stringent standards for product testing and purity. In a test from consumerlab.com, fish oils with little or no contamination included popular brands like Nordic Naturals, Pure Encapsulations, Carlson, and Kirkland.

Helpful: EPA- and DHA-containing algae supplements are a good option for vegetarians.

Polyphenols (OPCs and Curcumin)

As I discussed in Chapter 10, two plant compounds are uniquely effective depression fighters: oligomeric proanthocyanidins (OPCs), chemical compounds found in red grapes, blueberries, green tea, and other colorful plants and herbs; and curcumin, the active ingredient of the spice turmeric. There are no blood tests for OPCs, although tests that measure inflammation (like C-reactive protein, or CRP) can indicate whether your intake of anti-inflammatory, antioxidant OPCs is too low.

Supplementation

The best way to treat with OPCs is to use a combination rather than just one. The combined supplement I use in my practice is one I formulated: CurcumaSorb Mind, from Pure Encapsulations. It contains many of the OPCs discussed in Chapter 10, including grape extract, blueberry extract, green tea extract, and pine bark extract. It also contains curcumin.

Dose: CurcumaSorb Mind, two pills a day.

Timing: one with breakfast, one with dinner.

Important: If you decide to take curcumin separately, I recommend the well-studied (and well-absorbed) brands Theracurmin or Meriva. Research shows that Theracurmin is up to twenty-seven times more bioavailable than other curcumin supplements, and Meriva is up to twenty-nine times more bioavailable. Take Theracurmin at 60 to 180 mg per day, or Meriva at up to 500 to 2,000 mg per day.

Helpful: For maximum availability, take your curcumin supplement with or shortly after a meal or a snack.

Recapping the Plan

Here are the most important points to remember about the Antidepressant Deprescribing Plan—arguably the safest, most effective way to decrease or stop your use of antidepressants.

1. SSRIs/SNRIs have a profound effect on the way your brain functions.

2. They make serotonin bind to the serotonin receptors on the surface of neurons for longer periods of time—triggering your body to produce *less* serotonin.

3. When you stop taking the SSRI/SNRI, you go into a kind of serotonin shock from low levels of serotonin—with headaches, brain zaps, irritability, insomnia, intense agitation, and even suicidality.

4. But not *everybody* has withdrawal symptoms. On average, half of those stopping the drug have the symptoms and half don't.

5. Those with the worst symptoms have the most significant nutritional deficiencies.

6. That's because several nutrients—like zinc, vitamin D, folate, B6, and B12—are essential cofactors in the creation of serotonin.

7. If you're deficient in one of those nutrients, or you're genetically programmed with a need for higher levels of the nutrient, or your body is deficient in that nutrient—when you stop the SSRI/SNRI, and your body tries to produce more serotonin, it can't,

because it doesn't have the raw materials for serotonin production.

8. To safely deprescribe from SSRIs/SNRIs, you need to *test* for the levels of these nutrients, use targeted nutritional supplementation to correct low levels, and only *then* start your taper off your SSRI/SNRI.

9. Work in partnership with your doctor to do just that!

The Future of Happiness

> Nutritional therapies are an essential
> addition to psychological therapy in ending
> the epidemic of depression.

When they arrive at my office for the first time, many of my patients with depression are discouraged.

They're discouraged because they were assured by their previous doctors that medical treatment for depression would be effective—and it wasn't. They are discouraged because they are *still* depressed.

Most of these patients have tried at least one antidepressant medication. Some, as many as seven.

And although their individual stories differ, there is a common theme: a profound sense of having been let down by psychiatry.

It is for these discouraged people that I wrote this book.

I wrote it to give you *hope.*

I wrote it to give you *relief.*

I wrote it so you can have an alternative to a class of drugs that may not be working for you, or at least not working very well.

Yes, using the tests and treatments offered in this book, you can—*finally!*—free yourself from depressed moods.

New Treatments, New Hope

I've covered a lot in this book, looking at everything from free-form amino acids to zinc. And as I finish writing, I find myself asking the same types of questions that prompted me to write it in the first place. Questions like:

Research strongly links low levels of vitamin B12 and folate to depression. Why are vitamin B12 and folate levels not routinely checked in every patient who is depressed?

Deficiencies in trace minerals like zinc, magnesium, lithium, and chromium are also linked to depression. Why are so many psychiatrists reluctant to explore this link?

Why do health insurance companies routinely fail to cover nutritional supplements—even when lab tests reveal a nutritional deficiency?

The practice of Functional Psychiatry addresses these questions (and many more). It takes the link between nutrition and depression seriously, and it presents practical solutions.

Bottom line: Depressed patients should
receive effective help *now*.

Functional Psychiatry offers the know-how and the tools to correct the nutritional and metabolic factors that influence mood—the tools you'll find in this book.

I encourage you to engage your health professional in a broad search for the factors that may be contributing to your depression—and in correcting those factors.

You *can* find the help you need, and the peace of mind you deserve.

Depression is treatable. You *can* be hopeful. As I said in the beginning of the book, and I enthusiastically say again: the time for true healing is now.

More Resources

James Greenblatt, MD website

www.jamesgreenblattmd.com

This website is a source of information, support, and encouragement for those navigating mental illness, whether for yourself or a loved one. It includes:

- Web-based courses for consumers and professionals on topics ranging from depression to ADHD to anorexia nervosa and binge eating disorder.

- Descriptions of books by Dr. Greenblatt, and downloadable ebooks by Dr. Greenblatt.

- Articles by Dr. Greenblatt, covering a wide range of topics on using Functional Psychiatry for mental health and healing.

- Nutritional supplement protocols.

- Content incorporating materials from www.finallyfocused.com (on the ADHD book, *Finally Focused*).

- A provider directory of professionals in Functional Psychiatry.

- Links to websites that feature functional and integrative approaches to mental health.

- Information to contact Dr. Greenblatt.

Psychiatry Redefined website

www.psychiatryredefined.org

This website is an educational platform established to promote the advancement of Functional, Integrative, and Nutritional Psychiatry, and to provide health professionals with concept-to-application training in Functional Medicine for mental illness. The linked content of the website forms the foundation of the one-year Psychiatry Redefined Fellowship, a curriculum including more than thirty courses, fifty webinars, and numerous conference lectures. Fellows earn a Certificate of Training Completion, and are recognized as Psychiatry Redefined Certified Functional Medicine Providers—distinguishing graduates as leaders in the field of mental health care.

Several elements of the website are of potential interest to people who are not health professionals, including:

- a directory of mental health professionals trained in the Functional Medicine protocols of Psychiatry Redefined for depression, ADHD, obsessive-compulsive disorder (OCD), anorexia nervosa, and many other mental health issues;

- an archive of dozens of articles about Functional Psychiatry for mental health; and

- links to free webinars.

Books by James Greenblatt, MD

Dr. Greenblatt has authored many books dedicated to treating and resolving mental illness, and to establishing a new, biology-based paradigm for the treatment of mental illness. These books are featured on both james greenblattmd.com and psychiatryredefined.com. They include:

Functional Medicine for Antidepressant Withdrawal

Finally Focused: The Breakthrough Natural Treatment Plan for ADHD That Restores Attention, Minimizes Hyperactivity, and Helps Eliminate Drug Side Effects

Answers to Anorexia (second edition)

Integrative Medicine for Binge Eating

Brain Tonic: Your Healing Guide to the Revolutionary Neuro-Remedy, Low-Dose Nutritional Lithium

Integrative Medicine for Alzheimer's

Irritability and Anger: A Lithium Deficiency Disease? (ebook)

Irritability and Anger: The Role of Copper Toxicity (ebook)

Preventing Cognitive Decline and Dementia (ebook)

Action Plans

Amino Acids

Recommended Supplements

PRODUCT	IMPORTANCE	DOSING	NOTES
Amino Replete *Pure Encapsulations*	Balances neurotransmitters, often producing remarkable results—better mood and more energy—within weeks.	Take one scoop (4 g) twice daily in a glass of water or juice between meals.	Don't mix with a protein-rich liquid like yogurt or milk, which will decrease absorption.
Digestive Enzymes Ultra with Betaine HCl *Pure Encapsulations*	Ensures efficient protein digestion.	Take one to two capsules at the start of every meal: breakfast, lunch, and dinner.	You can find similar digestive enzyme/HCl formulations from other companies. Just make sure they contain Betaine HCl—the lack of this ingredient is the number one reason people on free-form amino acids and a digestive enzyme/HCl product don't experience improvement.
NeuroPure *Pure Encapsulations*	Boosts 5-HTP and phenylalanine, raising levels of serotonin and dopamine.	Take two capsules daily: one with breakfast, and one with dinner.	After one month, increase to two capsules with meals.
SeroPlus *Pure Encapsulations*	Raises levels of serotonin.	Take two capsules daily: one with breakfast, and one with dinner.	Helpful for antidepressant withdrawal tapering.

Possible Lab Tests

TEST PANEL	IMPORTANCE	COMPANY
ION Profile	This profile measures more than 150 biomarkers that provide insight into a patient's health. Common clinical indicators for ION testing include depression and other mood disorders, and digestive dysfunction.	Genova Diagnostics
Amino Acid Panel	This panel helps determine whether you have enough protein in your diet and whether the protein is properly digested and absorbed. Low levels indicate a need for supplementation.	Doctor's Data

Additional Information

- *Do not take NeuroPure or SeroPlus if you are on anti-depressants or have a history of bipolar illness.*

- For the Amino Acid Profile, pretest fasting is critical to ensure that test results are accurate, since food consumption influences amino acid levels.

- A free-form amino acid supplement supplies amino acids for four to five hours. Take the supplement at least twice per day, between meals.

Vitamin D

Recommended Supplements

PRODUCT	IMPORTANCE	DOSING	NOTES
Vitamin D3 & K2	Low levels of vitamin D are strongly linked to depression.	Take one capsule daily with food.	You can start taking vitamin D without laboratory testing, but testing is a must long-term. You will need to measure your blood level, and take a dosage that helps you boost vitamin D to an optimal level. Retest in sixty days.

Possible Lab Test

TEST PANEL	IMPORTANCE	COMPANY
Vitamin D *25-hydroxyvitamin D*	Severe deficiency: < 20 ng/mL Insufficiency: 20–30 ng/mL Low-normal: 30–40 ng/mL Optimal: 40–60 ng/mL	Quest/Labcorp

Additional Information

- When testing, it is important to test the storage form of Vitamin D: 25-hydroxy vitamin D. The active form (1,25-hydroxyvitamin D) is generally not considered to be an accurate marker.

- Vitamin D3 is safer than vitamin D2 and should be taken with vitamin K2.

- Once you have achieved optimal levels of vitamin D, I recommend you test levels twice per year to ensure levels stay in the optimal range—and increase your dosage if levels are low.

B Vitamins

Recommended Supplements

PRODUCT	IMPORTANCE	DOSING	NOTES
B-Complex Plus *Pure Encapsulations*	Low levels of many B vitamins—particularly folate and vitamin B12—play a role in depression.	Take one capsule, one to two times daily with food.	For thiamine supplementation—in fact, for getting a therapeutic, brain-healing dose of *all* the B vitamins—I recommend B-Complex Plus, from Pure Encapsulations. It supplies plenty of thiamine, riboflavin, niacin, vitamin B6, folate, vitamin B12, biotin, and pantothenic acid. If you've got a vitamin B12 or folate deficiency, you should add PureMelt B12 Folate.
PureMelt B12 Folate *Pure Encapsulations*		Dissolve one tablet in the mouth, one to two times daily.	
LMF		1–15 mg daily.	Begin with a dose of 1–3 mg daily and increase gradually, as needed.

Possible Lab Tests

TEST PANEL	IMPORTANCE	COMPANY
Serum B12	Low (< 150 nanograms per liter, or ng/L) and low-normal levels (< 600 ng/L) are indicative of potential deficiency or need for B12 supplementation. Normal levels (> 600 ng/L) *do not* rule out deficiency.	Quest/Labcorp
MMA	High levels (> 254 nmol/L) can indicate a deficiency or need for B12.	Quest/Labcorp
MTHFR Genetic Testing (C677T and A1298C variants)	Homozygous C677T (TT) and A1298C (CC) have increased requirements for LMF. Heterozygous C677T (CT) and A1298C (AC) often benefit from LMF supplementation as well.	Readily available from many testing laboratories
Homocysteine	High (> 12 µmol/L) can indicate a deficiency of B12 or folate.	Quest/Labcorp
2-Hydroxyhemopyrrolene-5-One (HPL)	High HPL levels indicate a need for vitamin B6 and zinc supplementation.	DHA Lab

Additional Information

- Include vitamin B12 in any supplement regimen that includes folate, to avoid masking B12 deficiency, which can cause nerve damage.

- Use a vitamin B6 supplement that is a fifty-fifty combination of pyridoxine and pyridoxal-5-phosphate (P5P, the active form of pyridoxine).

Minerals

Recommended Supplements

PRODUCT	IMPORTANCE	DOSING	NOTES
Trace Minerals	Zinc, chromium, iodine, and several other trace minerals are vital for brain health and in preventing and treating depression.	Take one capsule, one to two times daily with food.	A single trace mineral supplement can supply therapeutic doses of all the key trace minerals.
Zinc picolinate 15 mg		Take one to two capsules, twice daily with food.	Long-term use of zinc over 40 mg can cause copper deficiency. If you're taking zinc at that level, monitor copper levels and/or zinc levels. Dose should eventually be reduced to 15 mg, twice daily.
Magnesium Glycinate	Magnesium plays a role in hundreds of biochemical processes in the body, including in the brain, and is a must for supporting mental health.	Take 120 mg, three times daily: morning, afternoon, and before bed.	Magnesium relaxes muscles and nerves, and aids sleep.
Iron (ferrous bisglycinate)	Adequate iron is a must for mental health, and iron deficiency is linked to depression.	28 mg, once daily with a meal and a dose of vitamin C (see below).	This form of iron does not usually cause the typical side effects of iron supplementation, including constipation, nausea, and upset stomach.
Vitamin C	Vitamin C increases iron absorption.	250 mg (take at the same time with iron).	Consuming doses of 2,000 mg or more daily can cause upset stomach and diarrhea.

Possible Lab Test

TEST PANEL	IMPORTANCE	COMPANY
Trace Mineral Hair Analysis	This test helps identify mineral deficiencies and imbalances (like too much copper).	Doctor's Data

Additional Information

- Magnesium (particularly magnesium oxide) can sometimes cause loose stools. If you have this side effect, reduce the dose, switch to another type of magnesium (for example, to magnesium citrate or magnesium glycinate), and make sure you take the supplement with a meal.

Lithium Orotate

Recommended Supplement

PRODUCT	IMPORTANCE	DOSING	NOTES
Lithium orotate, 1 mg *Pure Encapsulations*	Low intake of this trace mineral is strongly linked to suicidality, irritability, and aggression.	Take 2 mg daily to start. Increase as needed in 5 mg increments (using the 5 mg product from Pure Encapsulations) to a total daily dose of up to 10 mg.	You can take low-dose nutritional lithium in the form of lithium orotate without testing. However, do not take more than 10 mg without the approval and supervision of a doctor familiar with the use of low-dose nutritional lithium.

Possible Lab Test

TEST PANEL	IMPORTANCE	COMPANY
Trace Mineral Hair Analysis	This test can help identify nutrient deficiencies or elevated copper and other toxicities.	Doctor's Data

Additional Information

- Don't take lithium orotate if you're trying to conceive, pregnant, or have kidney or thyroid disease.

EFAs

Recommended Supplements

PRODUCT	IMPORTANCE	DOSING	NOTES
Equazen Pro *SFI Health*	Omega-3 deficiencies are very common. But so are imbalances in omega-3 and omega-6 ratios. Equazen Pro provides a balanced ratio of omega-3s and omega-6s.	Three to six softgels daily.	Higher doses are used if testing shows a deficiency in EFAs.

Possible Lab Tests

TEST PANEL	IMPORTANCE	COMPANY
ION Profile	This profile measures more than 150 biomarkers that provide insight into a patient's health. Common clinical indications for ION testing include mood disorders and digestive dysfunction.	Genova Diagnostics
Fatty Acid Profile	An omega-6 to omega-3 ratio of two to one is ideal. Higher levels of omega-6 mean you need more omega-3.	Many labs offer a fatty acid profile.
Omega-3 Index	Low levels are indicative of a deficiency.	Quest

Additional Information

- While the body can convert plant-based ALA to EPA and DHA, the conversion is slow. And it depends on other nutritional factors, like zinc. That's why I favor direct consumption of EPA and DHA—through supplements and seafood—as the best way to normalize blood levels.

- Research shows that EPA has more mental health benefits than DHA. Look for a supplement with an EPA-to-DHA ratio greater than two-to-one.

- Because omega-3 deficiency is so prevalent, you can take up to 3,000 mg per day for as long as three months without testing.

Three months of daily omega-3 supplementation is often sufficient to correct a deficiency.

• Equazen Pro from SFI Health is my preferred fatty acid supplement. It is a clinically proven supplement that contains a balanced ratio of omega-3s *and* essential omega-6s. Omega-6
deficiency is often overlooked by practitioners

Polyphenols

Recommended Supplement

PRODUCT	IMPORTANCE	DOSING	NOTES
CurcumaSorb Mind *Pure Encapsulations*	Curcumin, the active ingredient in the spice turmeric, is a powerful anti-inflammatory and antioxidant, reducing the neuroinflammation that is linked to depression.	Take two capsules, one to three times daily between meals.	The OPCs found in green tea, red grapes, blueberries, and other colorful plants have a wide variety of brain-healing effects.

Additional Information

- The best way to treat with OPCs: Use a combination of OPCs rather than just one. The combined OPC supplement I use in my practice is one I formulated myself: CurcumaSorb Mind, from Pure Encapsulations. It contains many of the OPCs we've discussed in this book: grape extract, blueberry extract, green tea extract, and pine bark extract. It also contains curcumin.

ACKNOWLEDGMENTS

I would like to thank my wife, Judy, for her ongoing support, patience, and partnership; and my children, Julia and Nathan, my joy and inspiration.

To my parents, I extend a debt of gratitude for the lifetime of encouragement and support they have provided.

I would also like to thank:

Bill Gottlieb, my coauthor, with deep appreciation for the many years of our enjoyable and successful collaboration, and for his hard work, insight, and skill.

Scott Buesing, ND, for his astute and helpful review of the manuscript.

Jennifer Dimino, MS, for her ongoing research and assistance in all of my writing, lectures, and courses.

Josh Habansky, MSN, APRN, PMHNP-BC, a psychiatric nurse practitioner, for contributing several Functional Psychiatry case histories to this book.

Chris Tomasino, my literary agent, for her tireless support as she guides me through the publishing process, from proposal to bound book, and beyond.

NOTES

CHAPTER 1
Understanding Depression

1. "Major Depression," National Institute of Mental Health, https://www.nimh .nih.gov/health/statistics/major-depression.
2. Deborah S. Hasin et al., "Epidemiology of Adult *DSM-5* Major Depressive Disorder and Its Specifiers in the United States," *JAMA Psychiatry* 75, no. 4 (2018): 336–46, https://jamanetwork.com/journals/jamapsychiatry/fullarticle/2671413.
3. G. E. Simon and M. VonKorff, "Suicide Mortality Among Patients Treated for Depression in an Insured Population," *American Journal of Epidemiology* 147, no. 2 (January 15, 1998):155–60, https://pubmed.ncbi.nlm.nih.gov/9457005/.
4. "Suicide Statistics," American Foundation for Suicide Prevention, https://afsp .org/suicide-statistics/.
5. "Suicide and Self-Harm Injury," National Center for Health Statistics, Centers for Disease Control and Prevention, https://www.cdc.gov/nchs/fastats/suicide .htm.
6. Debra J. Brody et al., "Antidepressant Use Among Adults: United States, 2015–2018," NCHS Data Brief no. 377 (September 2020): https://www.cdc.gov/nchs /products/databriefs/db377.htm.
7. Crescent B. Martin et al., "Prescription Drug Use in the United States, 2015–2016," NCHS Data Brief no. 334 (May 2019): https://www.cdc.gov/nchs /products/databriefs/db334.htm.
8. Dekel Taliaz et al., "Optimizing Prediction of Response to Antidepressant Medications Using Machine Learning and Integrated Genetic, Clinical, and Demographic Data," *Translational Psychiatry* 11, no. 381 (2021): https://www.nature .com/articles/s41398-021-01488-3?utm.
9. Sidney Kennedy et al., "Pharmacotherapy to Sustain the Fully Remitted State," *Journal of Psychiatry and Neuroscience* 27, no. 4 (July 2002): 269–80, https:// pmc.ncbi.nlm.nih.gov/articles/PMC161661/.
10. Boris Voinov et al., "Depression and Chronic Diseases: It Is Time for a Synergistic Mental Health and Primary Care Approach," *The Primary Care Companion for CNS Disorders* 4, no. 15 (April 2013), https://pmc.ncbi.nlm.nih.gov/articles /PMC3733529.
11. "Persistent Depressive Disorder (Dysthymic Disorder)," National Institute of Mental Health, https://www.nimh.nih.gov/health/statistics/persistent-depressive -disorder-dysthymic-disorder.
12. "Seasonal Affective Disorder (SAD)," American Psychiatric Association, https:// www.psychiatry.org/patients-families/seasonal-affective-disorder.

13. PostpartumDepression.org, www.postpartumdepression.org.
14. Uriel Halbreich et al., "The Prevalence, Impairment, Impact, and Burden of Premenstrual Dysphoric Disorder (PMS/PMDD)," *Psychoneuroendocrinology* 28, Supplement 3 (August 2003): 1–23, https://pubmed.ncbi.nlm.nih.gov /12892987/.

CHAPTER 2
Psychiatry Redefined: The Future of Mental Healing Is Now

1. Allison Little, "Treatment-Resistant Depression," *American Family Physician* 80, no. 2 (2009): 167–172, https://www.aafp.org/pubs/afp/issues/2009/0715/p167 .html.
2. Nima Javadzade et al., "Effect of Mindfulness-Based Stress Reduction (MBSR) Program on Depression, Emotion Regulation, and Sleep Problems: A Randomized Controlled Trial Study on Depressed Elderly," *BMC Public Health* 24, no. 271 (2024), https://bmcpublichealth.biomedcentral.com/articles/10.1186 /s12889-024-17759-9.
3. Nate Cox et al., "Ketogenic Diets Potentially Reverse Type II Diabetes and Ameliorate Clinical Depression: A Case Study," *Diabetes & Metabolic Syndrome: Clinical Research & Reviews* 13, no. 2 (March–April 2019): 1475–79, https://www .sciencedirect.com/science/article/abs/pii/S1871402119300189.
4. Martha Rodríguez-Morán, "Combined Oral Supplementation with Magnesium Plus Vitamin D Alleviates Mild to Moderate Depressive Symptoms Related to Long-COVID: An Open-label Randomized, Controlled Clinical Trial," *Magnesium Research* 37, no. 3 (2024) https://pubmed.ncbi.nlm.nih.gov/39846976.
5. James S. Goodwin, "The Tomato Effect: Rejection of Highly Efficacious Therapies," *JAMA* 251, no. 18 (1984): 2387–90, https://jamanetwork.com/journals /jama/article-abstract/392749.

CHAPTER 4
Amino Acids: The Spark Plugs of Neurotransmission

1. H. C. Sabelli et al., "Phenylethylamine Modulation of Affect: Therapeutic and Diagnostic Implications," *The Journal of Neuropsychiatry and Clinical Neurosciences* 17, no. 1 (Winter 1995): 6–14, https://pubmed.ncbi.nlm.nih.gov /7711493/.
2. H. C. Sabelli, "Sustained Antidepressant Effect of PEA Replacement," *The Journal of Neuropsychiatry and Clinical Neurosciences* 8, no. 2 (May 1996): 168–71, https://psychiatryonline.org/doi/10.1176/jnp.8.2.168.
3. Purushottam Jangid et al., "Comparative Study of Efficacy of l-5-Hydroxytryptophan and Fluoxetine in Patients Presenting with First Depressive Episode," *Asian Journal of Psychiatry* 6, no. 1 (February 2013): 29–34, https:// pubmed.ncbi.nlm.nih.gov/23380314/.

CHAPTER 5
Vitamin D: *D* Is for Depression-Fighter

1. David O. Meltzer et al., "Association of Vitamin D Status and Other Clinical Characteristics With COVID-19 Test Results," *JAMA Network Open* 3, no. 9 (2020): https://jamanetwork.com/journals/jamanetworkopen/fullarticle /2770157.
2. Gaëlle Annweiler et al., "Vitamin D Supplementation Associated to Better Survival in Hospitalized Frail Elderly COVID-19 Patients: The GERIA-COVID Quasi-Experimental Study," *Nutrients* 11, no. 12 (2020): 3377, https://pubmed .ncbi.nlm.nih.gov/33147894/.
3. Xavier Nogues et al., "Calcifediol Treatment and COVID-19-Related Outcomes," *The Journal of Clinical Endocrinology and Metabolism* 106, no. 10 (September 27, 2021): e4017—e4027, https://pubmed.ncbi.nlm.nih.gov/34097036/.
4. Simon Spedding, "Vitamin D and Depression: A Systematic Review and Meta-Analysis Comparing Studies with and Without Biological Flaws," *Nutrients* 6, no. 4 (April 11, 2014):1501–18, https://pubmed.ncbi.nlm.nih.gov/24732019/.
5. Elizabeth R. Bertone-Johnson et al., "Vitamin D Intake from Foods and Supplements and Depressive Symptoms in a Diverse Population of Older Women," *American Journal of Clinical Nutrition*. 94, no. 4 (October 2011): 1104–12, https://pubmed.ncbi.nlm.nih.gov/21865327/.
6. Maria A. Polak et al., "Serum 25-Hydroxyvitamin D Concentrations and Depressive Symptoms Among Young Adult Men and Women," *Nutrients* 6, no. 11 (October 28, 2014): 4720–30, https://pmc.ncbi.nlm.nih.gov/articles/PMC 4245559.
7. Lucinda J. Black et al., "Low Vitamin D Levels Are Associated with Symptoms of Depression in Young Adult Males," *The Australian and New Zealand Journal of Psychiatry*. 48, no. 5 (May 2014): 464–71, https://pubmed.ncbi.nlm.nih.gov /24226892/.
8. Masha Omidian et al., "Effects of Vitamin D Supplementation on Depressive Symptoms in Type 2 Diabetes Mellitus Patients: Randomized Placebo-Controlled Double-Blind Clinical Trial," *Diabetes & Metabolic Syndrome: Clinical Research & Reviews* 13, no. 4 (July–August 2019): 2375–80, https://www .sciencedirect.com/science/article/abs/pii/S1871402119303236.
9. MinhTu T. Hoang et al., "Association Between Low Serum 25-Hydroxyvitamin D and Depression in a Large Sample of Healthy Adults: The Cooper Center Longitudinal Study," *Mayo Clinic Proceedings* 86, no. 11 (November 2011): 1050–5, https://pubmed.ncbi.nlm.nih.gov/22033249/.
10. Ying Chih Cheng et al., "The Effect of Vitamin D Supplement on Negative Emotions: A Systematic Review and Meta-Analysis," *Depression and Anxiety* 37, no. 6 (June 2020): 549–64, https://pubmed.ncbi.nlm.nih.gov/32365423/.
11. A. T. Lansdowne et al., "Vitamin D3 Enhances Mood in Healthy Subjects During Winter," *Psychopharmacology* 135, no. 4 (February 1998): 319–23, https:// pubmed.ncbi.nlm.nih.gov/9539254/.

12. Sun-Young Kim et al., "Vitamin D Deficiency and Suicidal Ideation: A Cross-Sectional Study of 157,211 Healthy Adults," *Journal of Psychosomatic Research* 134 (July 2020): 110125, https://pubmed.ncbi.nlm.nih.gov/32388454/.

13. Cécile Grudet et al., "Suicidal Patients Are Deficient in Vitamin D, Associated with a Pro-Inflammatory Status in the Blood," *Psychoneuroendocrinology* 50 (December 2014): 210–19, https://pubmed.ncbi.nlm.nih.gov/25240206/.

14. Gamze Gokalp, "The Association Between Low Vitamin D Levels and Suicide Attempts in Adolescents," *Annals of Clinical Psychiatry* 32, no. 2 (May 2020): 106–13, https://pubmed.ncbi.nlm.nih.gov/32384132/.

15. Y. Milaneschi et al., "The Association Between Low Vitamin D and Depressive Disorders," *Molecular Psychiatry* 19, no. 4 (April 2014): 444–51, https://pubmed.ncbi.nlm.nih.gov/23568194/.

16. Greta Snellman et al., "Seasonal Genetic Influence on Serum 25-Hydroxyvitamin D Levels: A Twin Study," *PLoS One* 13, no. 4 (November 13, 2009): e7747, https://pubmed.ncbi.nlm.nih.gov/19915719/.

CHAPTER 6
B Vitamins: Building Blocks of a Better Brain

1. Henning Tiemeier et al., "Vitamin B12, Folate, and Homocysteine in Depression: The Rotterdam Study," *American Journal of Psychiatry* 159, no. 12 (December 2002): 2099–101, https://pubmed.ncbi.nlm.nih.gov/12450964/.

2. Jukka Hintikka et al., "High Vitamin B12 Level and Good Treatment Outcome May Be Associated in Major Depressive Disorder," *BMC Psychiatry* 3, no. 17 (December 2, 2003), https://pubmed.ncbi.nlm.nih.gov/14641930/.

3. Yongjun Tan et al., "Vitamin B12, Folate, Homocysteine, Inflammatory Mediators (Interleukin-6, Tumor Necrosis Factor-α and C-Reactive Protein) Levels in Adolescents with Anxiety or Depressive Symptoms," *Neuropsychiatric Disease and Treatment* 19 (April 7, 2023): 785–800, https://pubmed.ncbi.nlm.nih.gov/37056916/.

4. Yanjun Wu et al., "Associations of Dietary B Vitamins Intakes with Depression in Adults," *International Journal of Vitamin and Nutrition Research* 93, no. 2 (April 2023): 142–53, https://pubmed.ncbi.nlm.nih.gov/34233510/.

5. Jaqueline G. Borges-Vieira et al., "Efficacy of B-Vitamins and Vitamin D Therapy in Improving Depressive and Anxiety Disorders: A Systematic Review of Randomized Controlled Trials," *Nutritional Neuroscience* 26, no. 3 (March 2023): 187–207, https://pubmed.ncbi.nlm.nih.gov/35156551/.

6. Yiqi Wang et al., "Associations Between Dietary Intake, Diet Quality and Depressive Symptoms in Youth: A Systematic Review of Observational Studies," *Health Promotion Perspectives* 12, no. 3 (December 10, 2022): 249–65, https://pubmed.ncbi.nlm.nih.gov/36686054/.

7. Josué Cruz-Rodríguez et al., "Association Between of Vitamin B12 Status During Pregnancy and Probable Postpartum Depression: The ECLIPSES Study," *Journal*

of Reproductive and Infant Psychology (March 5, 2024): 1–15, https://pubmed.ncbi.nlm.nih.gov/38440867/.

8. Jie Li et al., Association Between Suicide Attempts and Anemia in Late-Life Depression Inpatients," *BMC Geriatrics* (January 10, 2024): 24–43, https://pmc.ncbi.nlm.nih.gov/articles/PMC10782764/.

9. Yongjun Tan et al., "Correlation Between Vitamin B12 and Mental Health in Children and Adolescents: A Systematic Review and Meta-Analysis," *Clinical Psychopharmacology and Neuroscience* 21, no. 4 (June 2, 2023): 617–33, https://pmc.ncbi.nlm.nih.gov/articles/PMC10591166/.

10. Ibrahim Elmadfa et al., "Vitamin B-12 and Homocysteine Status Among Vegetarians: A Global Perspective," *American Journal of Clinical Nutrition* 89, no. 5 (May 2009): 1693S—98S, https://pubmed.ncbi.nlm.nih.gov/19357223/.

11. Natasha Kate et al., "Does B12 Deficiency Lead to Lack of Treatment Response to Conventional Antidepressants?," *Psychiatry* 7, no. 11 (November 2010): 42–44, https://pmc.ncbi.nlm.nih.gov/articles/PMC3010969/.

12. A. David Smith et al., "Homocysteine and Dementia: An International Consensus Statement," *Journal of Alzheimer's Disease* 62, no. 2 (2018): 561–70, https://pubmed.ncbi.nlm.nih.gov/29480200/.

13. Sebastian Ocklenburg et al., "Vegetarian Diet and Depression Scores: A Meta-Analysis," *Journal of Affective Disorders* 294 (November 1, 2021): 813–15, https://pubmed.ncbi.nlm.nih.gov/34375207/.

14. Ansley Bender et al., "The Association of Folate and Depression: A Meta-Analysis," *Journal of Psychiatric Analysis* 95 (December 2017): 9–18, https://pubmed.ncbi.nlm.nih.gov/28759846/.

15. Marisa I. Ramos et al., "Plasma Folate Concentrations Are Associated with Depressive Symptoms in Elderly Latina Women Despite Folic Acid Fortification," *American Journal of Clinical Nutrition* 80, no. 4 (October 2004): 1024–28, https://pubmed.ncbi.nlm.nih.gov/15447915/.

16. George I. Papakostas et al., "L-Methylfolate as Adjunctive Therapy for SSRI-Resistant Major Depression: Results of Two Randomized, Double-Blind, Parallel-Sequential Trials," *American Journal of Psychiatry* 169, no. 12 (December 2012): 1267–74, https://pubmed.ncbi.nlm.nih.gov/23212058/.

17. Richard C. Shelton et al., "Assessing Effects of l-Methylfolate in Depression Management: Results of a Real-World Patient Experience Trial," *The Primary Care Companion for CNS Disorders* 15, no. 4 (August 29, 2013): https://pubmed.ncbi.nlm.nih.gov/24392264/.

18. Vladimir Maletic et al., "A Review of l-Methylfolate as Adjunctive Therapy in the Treatment of Major Depressive Disorder," *The Primary Care Companion for CNS Disorders* 25, no. 3 (May 9, 2023): https://pubmed.ncbi.nlm.nih.gov/37192264/.

19. Abdullah Al Maruf et al., "Systematic Review and Meta-Analysis of L-Methylfolate Augmentation in Depressive Disorders," *Pharmacopsychiatry* 55, no. 3 (May 2022): 139–47, https://pubmed.ncbi.nlm.nih.gov/34794190/.

20. J. Brozek et al., "Psychological Effects of Thiamine Restriction and Deprivation

in Normal Young Men," *American Journal of Clinical Nutrition* 5, no. 2 (March–April 1957): 109–20, https://pubmed.ncbi.nlm.nih.gov/13410810/.

21. Geng Zhang et al., "Thiamine Nutritional Status and Depressive Symptoms Are Inversely Associated Among Older Chinese Adults," *The Journal of Nutrition* 1, no. 143 (January 2013): 53–58, https://pubmed.ncbi.nlm.nih.gov /23173173/.

22. Gary E. Gibson et al., "Pharmacological Thiamine Levels as a Therapeutic Approach in Alzheimer's Disease," *Frontiers in Medicine* 9 (October 4, 2022): 1033272, https://pmc.ncbi.nlm.nih.gov/articles/PMC9585656/.

23. D. Benton et al., "Vitamin Supplementation for 1 Year Improves Mood," *Neuropsychobiology* 32, no. 2 (1995): 98–105, https://pubmed.ncbi.nlm.nih.gov /7477807/.

24. L. J. Smidt et al., "Influence of Thiamin Supplementation on the Health and General Well-Being of an Elderly Irish Population with Marginal Thiamin Deficiency," *Journal of Gerontology* 46, no. 1 (January 1991): M16–22, https:// pubmed.ncbi.nlm.nih.gov/1986037/.

25. D. Benton et al., "Thiamine Supplementation Mood and Cognitive Functioning," *Psychopharmacology* 129 (1997): 66–71, https://pubmed.ncbi.nlm.nih.gov /9122365/.

26. Wu et al., "Associations of Dietary B Vitamins Intakes with Depression in Adults."

27. Yoonji Kim et al., "Association of the Anxiety/Depression with Nutrition Intake in Stroke Patients," *Clinical Nutrition Research* 7, no. 1 (January 2018): 11–20, https://pubmed.ncbi.nlm.nih.gov/29423385/.

28. Bo H. Jonsson, "Nicotinic Acid Long-Term Effectiveness in a Patient with Bipolar Type II Disorder: A Case of Vitamin Dependency," *Nutrients* 10, no. 2 (January 27, 2018): 134, https://pubmed.ncbi.nlm.nih.gov/29382049/.

CHAPTER 7
Minerals: Key Elements of Mental Well-Being

1. David Thomas, "The Mineral Depletion of Foods Available to Us as a Nation (1940–2002)—a Review of the 6th Edition of McCance and Widdowson," *Nutrition and Health* 19, no. 1–2 (2007): 21–55, https://pubmed.ncbi.nlm.nih.gov /18309763/.

2. Khanrin Phungamla Vashum et al., "Dietary Zinc Is Associated with a Lower Incidence of Depression: Findings from Two Australian Cohorts," *Journal of Affective Disorders* 166 (September 2014): 249–57, https://pubmed.ncbi.nlm.nih.gov /25012438/.

3. Marcin Siwek et al., "Serum Zinc Level in Depressed Patients During Zinc Supplementation of Imipramine Treatment," *Journal of Affective Disorders* 126, no. 3 (November 2010): 447–52, https://pubmed.ncbi.nlm.nih.gov/20493532/.

4. Falah S. Al-Fartusie et al., "Evaluation of Some Trace Elements and Vitamins in

Major Depressive Disorder Patients: A Case-Control Study," *Biological Trace Element Research* 189, no. 2 (June 2019): 412–19, https://pubmed.ncbi.nlm.nih.gov/30238421/.

5. T. Sawada et al., "Effect of Zinc Supplementation on Mood States in Young Women: A Pilot Study," *European Journal of Clinical Nutrition* 64 (January 20, 2010): 331–33, https://pubmed.ncbi.nlm.nih.gov/20087376/.

6. Somaye Yosaee et al., "Effects of Zinc, Vitamin D, and Their Co-Supplementation on Mood, Serum Cortisol, and Brain-Derived Neurotrophic Factor in Patients with Obesity and Mild to Moderate Depressive Symptoms," *Nutrition* 71 (March 2020): 71:110601, https://pubmed.ncbi.nlm.nih.gov/31837640/.

7. Soheila Salari et al., "Zinc Sulphate: A Reasonable Choice for Depression Management in Patients with Multiple Sclerosis: A Randomized, Double-Blind, Placebo-Controlled Clinical Trial," *Pharmacological Reports* 67, no. 3 (June 2015): https://pubmed.ncbi.nlm.nih.gov/25933976/.

8. Jun Lai et al., "The Efficacy of Zinc Supplementation in Depression: Systematic Review of Randomised Controlled Trials," *Journal of Affective Disorders* 136, no. 1–2, (January 2012): e31–e39, https://pubmed.ncbi.nlm.nih.gov/21798601/.

9. Krzysztof Styczén et al., "The Serum Zinc Concentration as a Potential Biological Marker in Patients with Major Depressive Disorder," *Metabolic Brain Disease* 32, no. 1 (August 8, 2016): 97–103, https://pubmed.ncbi.nlm.nih.gov/27502410/.

10. Jinhua Chen et al., "The Emerging Role of Copper in Depression," *Frontiers in Neuroscience* 17 (August 7, 2023): 17:1230404, https://pubmed.ncbi.nlm.nih.gov/37609453/.

11. Mengmei Ni et al., "Copper in Depressive Disorder: A Systematic Review and Meta-Analysis of Observational Studies," *Psychiatry Research* 267 (September 2018): 506–15, https://pubmed.ncbi.nlm.nih.gov/29980131/.

12. Saad Atiq et al., "A Unique Case of Severe Anemia Secondary to Copper Deficiency in an Adult Patient," *Cureus* 10, no. 11 (November 26, 2018): e3636, https://pubmed.ncbi.nlm.nih.gov/30723637/.

13. Bingrong Li et al., "Dietary Magnesium and Calcium Intake and Risk of Depression in the General Population: A Meta-Analysis," *The Australian and New Zealand Journal of Psychiatry* 51, no. 3 (March 2017): 219–29, https://pubmed.ncbi.nlm.nih.gov/27807012/.

14. Andrea Botturi et al., "The Role and the Effect of Magnesium in Mental Disorders: A Systematic Review," *Nutrients* 3, no. 12 (June 3, 2020): 1661, https://pubmed.ncbi.nlm.nih.gov/32503201/.

15. Mahdi Moabedi et al., "Magnesium Supplementation Beneficially Affects Depression in Adults with Depressive Disorder: A Systematic Review and Meta-Analysis of Randomized Clinical Trials," *Frontiers in Psychiatry* 14 (December 22, 2023): 1333261, https://pubmed.ncbi.nlm.nih.gov/38213402/.

16. Tapash Roy et al., "Epidemiology of Depression and Diabetes: A Systematic Re-

view," *Journal of Affective Disorders* 142 Suppl. (October 2012): S8–S21, https://pubmed.ncbi.nlm.nih.gov/23062861/.

17. Lazaro Barragán-Rodríguez et al., "Efficacy and Safety of Oral Magnesium Supplementation in the Treatment of Depression in the Elderly with Type 2 Diabetes: A Randomized, Equivalent Trial," *Magnesium Research* 21, no. 4 (December 2008): 218–23, https://pubmed.ncbi.nlm.nih.gov/19271419/.

18. Nadia Iovieno et al., "Second-Tier Natural Antidepressants: Review and Critique," *Journal of Affective Disorders* 130, no. 3 (May 2011): 343–57, https://pubmed.ncbi.nlm.nih.gov/20579741/.

19. Kimberly A. Brownley et al., "Dietary Chromium Supplementation for Targeted Treatment of Diabetes Patients with Comorbid Depression and Binge Eating," *Medical Hypotheses* 85, no. 1 (July 2015): 45–48, https://pubmed.ncbi.nlm.nih.gov/25838140/.

20. Malcolm N. McLeod et al., "Chromium Treatment of Depression," *International Journal of Neuropsychopharmacology* 3, no. 4 (December 2000): 311–14, https://pubmed.ncbi.nlm.nih.gov/11343609/.

21. Kimberly A. Brownley et al., "Chromium Supplementation for Menstrual Cycle-Related Mood Symptoms," *Journal of Dietary Supplements* 10, no. 4 (December 2013): 345–56, https://pubmed.ncbi.nlm.nih.gov/24237190/.

22. M. N. McLeod et al., "Chromium Potentiation of Antidepressant Pharmacotherapy for Dysthymic Disorder in 5 Patients," *Journal of Clinical Psychiatry* 60, no. 4 (April 1999): 237–40, https://pubmed.ncbi.nlm.nih.gov/10221284/.

23. Jonathan R. T. Davidson et al., "Effectiveness of Chromium in Atypical Depression: A Placebo-Controlled Trial," *Biological Psychiatry* 53, no. 3 (February 1, 2003): 261–64, https://pubmed.ncbi.nlm.nih.gov/12559660/.

24. John P. Docherty et al., "A Double-Blind, Placebo-Controlled, Exploratory Trial of Chromium Picolinate in Atypical Depression: Effect on Carbohydrate Craving," *Journal of Psychiatric Practice* 11, no. 5 (September 2005): 302–14, https://pubmed.ncbi.nlm.nih.gov/16184071/.

25. Henry Bode et al., "Hyperthyroidism and Clinical Depression: A Systematic Review and Meta-Analysis," *Translational Psychiatry* 12, no. 1 (September 5, 2022): 362, https://pubmed.ncbi.nlm.nih.gov/36064836/.

26. M. Bauer et al., "Role of Thyroid Hormone Therapy in Depressive Disorders," *Journal of Endocrinological Investigation* 44, no. 11 (November 2021): 2341–47, https://pubmed.ncbi.nlm.nih.gov/34129186/.

27. M. Vahdat Shariatpanaahi et al., "The Relationship Between Depression and Serum Ferritin Level," *European Journal of Clinical Nutrition* 61, no. 4 (April 2007): 532–35, https://pubmed.ncbi.nlm.nih.gov/17063146.

28. John L. Beard et al., "Maternal Iron Deficiency Anemia Affects Postpartum Emotions and Cognition," *Journal of Nutrition* 135, no. 2 (February 2005): 267–72, https://pubmed.ncbi.nlm.nih.gov/15671224/.

29. Zongyao Li et al., "Dietary Zinc and Iron Intake and Risk of Depression: A Meta-Analysis," *Psychiatry Research* 251 (May 2017): 41–47, https://pubmed.ncbi.nlm.nih.gov/28189077/.

CHAPTER 8
Low-Dose Nutritional Lithium:
Lowering the Risk of Suicide, Worldwide

1. Anjum Memon et al., "Association Between Naturally Occurring Lithium in Drinking Water and Suicide Rates: Systematic Review and Meta-Analysis of Ecological Studies," *British Journal of Psychiatry* 217, no. 6 (December 2020): 667–78, https://pubmed.ncbi.nlm.nih.gov/32716281/.

2. Johanna Wallensten et al., "Stress, Depression, and Risk of Dementia—a Cohort Study in the Total Population Between 18 and 65 Years Old in Region Stockholm," *Alzheimer's Research & Therapy* 15, no. 1 (October 2, 2023): 161, https://pubmed.ncbi.nlm.nih.gov/37779209/.

3. Tobias Gerhard et al., "Lithium Treatment and Risk for Dementia in Adults with Bipolar Disorder: Population-Based Cohort Study," *British Journal of Psychiatry*, no. 1 (July 2015): 46–51, https://pubmed.ncbi.nlm.nih.gov/25614530/.

4. Lars Vedel Kessing et al., "Lithium Treatment and Risk of Dementia," *Archives of General Psychiatry* 65, no. 11 (November 2008): 1331–35, https://pubmed.ncbi.nlm.nih.gov/18981345/.

5. Qiuying Lu et al., "Lithium Therapy's Potential to Lower Dementia Risk and the Prevalence of Alzheimer's Disease: A Meta-Analysis," *European Neurology* 87, no. 2 (2024): 93–104, https://pubmed.ncbi.nlm.nih.gov/38657568/.

6. Orestes V. Forlenza et al., "Disease-Modifying Properties of Long-Term Lithium Treatment for Amnestic Mild Cognitive Impairment: Randomised Controlled Trial," *British Journal of Psychiatry* 198, no. 5 (May 2011): 351–56, https://pubmed.ncbi.nlm.nih.gov/21525519/.

7. Orestes V. Forlenza et al., "Clinical and Biological Effects of Long-Term Lithium Treatment in Older Adults with Amnestic Mild Cognitive Impairment: Randomized Clinical Trial," *British Journal of Psychiatry* 215, no. 5 (November 2019): 668–74, https://pubmed.ncbi.nlm.nih.gov/30947755/.

8. Lars Vedel Kessing et al., "Association of Lithium in Drinking Water with the Incidence of Dementia," *JAMA Psychiatry* 74, no. 10 (October 1, 2017): 1005–10, https://pubmed.ncbi.nlm.nih.gov/28832877/.

9. Val Andrew Fajardo et al., "Examining the Relationship Between Trace Lithium in Drinking Water and the Rising Rates of Age-Adjusted Alzheimer's Disease Mortality in Texas," *Journal of Alzheimer's Disease* 61, no. 1 (2018): 425–34, https://pubmed.ncbi.nlm.nih.gov/29103043/.

10. Michael Ray Dickerson et al., "Pharmacogenetic Testing May Benefit People Receiving Low-Dose Lithium in Clinical Practice," *Journal of the American Association of Nurse Practitioners* 36, no. 6 (2024): 320–28, https://pubmed.ncbi.nlm.nih.gov/37882688/.

11. Rebecca Strawbridge et al., "Identifying the Neuropsychiatric Health Effects of Low-Dose Lithium Interventions: A Systematic Review," *Neuroscience and Biobe-*

havioral Reviews 144 (January 2023): 104975, https://pubmed.ncbi.nlm.nih
.gov/36436738/.

12. Timothy S. Murbach et al., "A Toxicological Evaluation of Lithium Orotate," *Regulatory Toxicology and Pharmacology* 124 (August 2021): 104973, https://pubmed.ncbi.nlm.nih.gov/34146638/.

CHAPTER 9
Essential Fats, Essential Healing

1. Christos F. Kelaiditis et al., "Effects of Long-Chain Omega-3 Polyunsaturated Fatty Acids on Reducing Anxiety and/or Depression in Adults: A Systematic Review and Meta-Analysis of Randomised Controlled Trials," *Prostaglandins, Leukotrienes, and Essential Fatty Acids* 192 (May 2023): 102572, https://pubmed.ncbi.nlm.nih.gov/37028202/.

2. Yuhua Liao et al., "Efficacy of Omega-3 PUFAs in Depression: A Meta-Analysis," *Translational Psychiatry* 9, no. 1 (August 5, 2019): 190, https://pubmed.ncbi.nlm.nih.gov/31383846/.

3. Stefania Lamon-Fava et al., "Clinical Response to EPA Supplementation in Patients with Major Depressive Disorder Is Associated with Higher Plasma Concentrations of Pro-Resolving Lipid Mediators," *Neuropsychopharmacology* 48, no. 6 (May 2023): 929–35, https://pubmed.ncbi.nlm.nih.gov/36635595/.

4. Yoko Nagayasu et al., "Possible Prevention of Post-Partum Depression by Intake of Omega-3 Polyunsaturated Fatty Acids and Its Relationship with Interleukin 6," *Journal of Obstetrics and Gynaecology Research* 47, no. 4 (April 2021): 1371–79, https://pubmed.ncbi.nlm.nih.gov/33590576/.

5. M. E. Berger et al., "Omega-6 to Omega-3 Polyunsaturated Fatty Acid Ratio and Subsequent Mood Disorders in Young People with At-Risk Mental States: A 7-Year Longitudinal Study," *Translational Psychiatry* 7, no. 8 (August 29, 2017): e1220, https://pubmed.ncbi.nlm.nih.gov/28850110/.

6. Joseph R. Hibbeln et al., "The Potential for Military Diets to Reduce Depression, Suicide, and Impulsive Aggression: A Review of Current Evidence for Omega-3 and Omega-6 Fatty Acids," *Military Medicine* 179, no. 11 Suppl. (November 2014): 117–28, https://pubmed.ncbi.nlm.nih.gov/25373095/.

7. Michael D. Lewis et al., "Suicide Deaths of Active Duty U.S. Military and Omega-3 Fatty Acid Status: A Case Control Comparison," *Journal of Clinical Psychiatry* 72, no. 12 (December 2011): 1585–90, https://pubmed.ncbi.nlm.nih.gov/21903029/.

8. Helena Sofia Antao et al., "Omega-3 Index as Risk Factor in Psychiatric Diseases: A Narrative Review," *Frontiers in Psychiatry* 14 (July 28, 2023): 1200403, https://pubmed.ncbi.nlm.nih.gov/37575565/.

9. R. E. Morgan et al., "Plasma Cholesterol and Depressive Symptoms in Older Men," *Lancet* 341, no. 8837 (January 9, 1993): 75–79, https://pubmed.ncbi.nlm.nih.gov/8093404/.

10. P. H. Steegmans et al., "Higher Prevalence of Depressive Symptoms in Middle-Aged Men with Low Serum Cholesterol Levels," *Psychosomatic Medicine* 62, no. 2 (March–April 2000): 205–11, https://pubmed.ncbi.nlm.nih.gov /10772398/.

11. M. Horsten et al., "Depressive Symptoms, Social Support, and Lipid Profile in Healthy Middle-Aged Women," *Psychosomatic Medicine* 59, no. 5 (September–October 1997): 521–28, https://pubmed.ncbi.nlm.nih.gov/9316185/.

12. Joseph A. Boscarino et al., "Low Serum Cholesterol and External-Cause Mortality: Potential Implications for Research and Surveillance," *Journal of Psychiatric Research* 43, no. 9 (June 2009): 848–54, https://pubmed.ncbi.nlm.nih.gov /19135214/.

13. D. Rafter, "Biochemical Markers of Anxiety and Depression," *Psychiatry Research* 103, no. 1 (August 5, 2001): 93–96, https://pubmed.ncbi.nlm.nih.gov /11472794/.

14. Ju Young Shin et al., "Are Cholesterol and Depression Inversely Related? A Meta-Analysis of the Association Between Two Cardiac Risk Factors," *Annals of Behavioral Medicine* 36, no. 1 (August 2008): 33–43, https://pubmed.ncbi.nlm.nih .gov/18787911/.

15. Soili M. Lehto et al., "Low Serum HDL-Cholesterol Levels Are Associated with Long Symptom Duration in Patients with Major Depressive Disorder," *Psychiatry and Clinical Neurosciences* 64, no. 3 (June 2010): 279–83, https://pubmed.ncbi .nlm.nih.gov/20374538/.

16. Maja Vilibić et al., "Association Between Total Serum Cholesterol and Depression, Aggression, and Suicidal Ideations in War Veterans with Posttraumatic Stress Disorder: A Cross-Sectional Study," *Croatian Medical Journal* 55, no. 5 (October 2014): 520–29, https://pubmed.ncbi.nlm.nih.gov/25358885/.

17. Chu-Chiao Tseng et al., "High-Density Lipoprotein Cholesterol Abnormalities Correlate with Severe Fatigue in Major Depressive Disorder: A Cross-Sectional Study," *Journal of Psychosomatic Research* 184 (September 2024): 111835, https:// pubmed.ncbi.nlm.nih.gov/39002265/.

CHAPTER 10
Polyphenols: Powerful Phytochemicals in Plants and Foods

1. Jessica Bayes et al., "Effects of Polyphenols in a Mediterranean Diet on Symptoms of Depression: A Systematic Literature Review," *Advances in Nutrition* 11, no. 3 (May 1, 2020): 602–15, https://pubmed.ncbi.nlm.nih.gov/31687743/.

2. Jeanne Bardinet et al., "Patterns of Polyphenol Intake and Risk of Depressive Symptomatology in a Population-Based Cohort of Older Adults," *Clinical Nutrition* 41, no. 12 (December 2022): 2628–36, https://pubmed.ncbi.nlm.nih.gov /36308981/.

3. Jay Jay Thaung Zaw et al., "Long-Term Resveratrol Supplementation Improves Pain Perception, Menopausal Symptoms, and Overall Well-Being in Postmeno-

pausal Women: Findings from a 24-Month Randomized, Controlled, Crossover Trial," *Menopause* 28, no. 1 (August 31, 2020): 40–49, https://pubmed.ncbi .nlm.nih.gov/32881835/.

4. Samira Menegas et al., "Potential Mechanisms of Action of Resveratrol in Prevention and Therapy for Mental Disorders," *Journal of Nutritional Biochemistry* 121 (November 2023): 109435, https://pubmed.ncbi.nlm.nih.gov/37669710/.

5. Gioacchino Calapai et al., "A Randomized, Double-Blinded, Clinical Trial on Effects of a *Vitis vinifera* Extract on Cognitive Function in Healthy Older Adults," *Frontiers in Pharmacology* 8 (October 31, 2017: 776, https://pubmed.ncbi.nlm .nih.gov/29163162/.

6. Masakazu Terauchi et al., "Effects of Grape Seed Proanthocyanidin Extract on Menopausal Symptoms, Body Composition, and Cardiovascular Parameters in Middle-Aged Women: A Randomized, Double-Blind, Placebo-Controlled Pilot Study," *Menopause* 21, no. 9 (September 2014): 990–96, https://pubmed.ncbi .nlm.nih.gov/24518152/.

7. Jonathan Sinclair et al., "Effects of Montmorency Tart Cherry and Blueberry Juice on Cardiometabolic and Other Health-Related Outcomes: A Three-Arm Placebo Randomized Controlled Trial," *International Journal of Environmental Research and Public Health* 19, no. 9 (April 27, 2022): 5317, https://pubmed .ncbi.nlm.nih.gov/35564709/.

8. Yekta Dowlati et al., "Selective Dietary Supplementation in Early Postpartum Is Associated with High Resilience Against Depressed Mood," *Proceedings of the National Academy of Sciences* 114, no. 13 (March 28, 2017): 3509–14, https:// pubmed.ncbi.nlm.nih.gov/28289215/.

9. Robert Krikorian et al., "Blueberry Supplementation Improves Memory in Older Adults," *Journal of Agricultural and Food Chemistry* 58, no. 7 (April 14, 2010): 3996–4000, https://pubmed.ncbi.nlm.nih.gov/20047325/.

10. Sundus Khalid et al., "Effects of Acute Blueberry Flavonoids on Mood in Children and Young Adults," *Nutrients* 9, no. 2 (February 20, 2017): 158, https:// pubmed.ncbi.nlm.nih.gov/28230732/.

11. Akinori Yaegashi et al., "Green Tea Consumption and Risk of Depression Symptoms: A Systematic Review and Meta-Analysis of Observational Studies," *Journal of Nutritional Science and Vitaminology* 68, no. 3 (2022): 155–61, https:// pubmed.ncbi.nlm.nih.gov/35768246/.

12. T. P. Ng et al., "Tea Consumption and Depression from Follow Up in the Singapore Longitudinal Ageing Study," *Journal of Nutrition, Health, & Aging* 25, no. 3 (2021): 295–301, https://pubmed.ncbi.nlm.nih.gov/33575719/.

13. Agnieszka Micek et al., "Polyphenol-Rich Beverages and Mental Health Outcomes," *Antioxidants* 12, no. 2 (January 25, 2023): 272, https://pubmed.ncbi .nlm.nih.gov/36829831/.

14. Dehghan Manshadi Seyed Ali et al., "Effect of Green Tea Consumption in Treatment of Mild to Moderate Depression in Iranian Patients Living with HIV: A Double-Blind Randomized Clinical Trial," *Chinese Herbal Medicines* 13, no. 1 (November 26, 2020): 136–41, https://pubmed.ncbi.nlm.nih.gov/36117757/.

15. Shinsuke Hidese et al., "Effects of Chronic L-Theanine Administration in Patients with Major Depressive Disorder: An Open-Label Study," *Acta Neuropsychiatrica* 29, no. 2 (April 2017): 72–79, https://pubmed.ncbi.nlm.nih.gov /27396868/.

16. Ahmad Shamabadi et al., "L-Theanine Adjunct to Sertraline for Major Depressive Disorder: A Randomized, Double-Blind, Placebo-Controlled Clinical Trial," *Journal of Affective Disorders* 333 (July 15, 2023): 38–43, https://pubmed.ncbi .nlm.nih.gov/37084960/.

17. Keiko Unno et al., "Improvement of Depressed Mood with Green Tea Intake," *Nutrients* 14, no. 14 (July 19, 2022): 2949, https://pubmed.ncbi.nlm.nih.gov /35889906/.

18. Jie Shao et al., "A Comprehensive Review on Bioavailability, Safety and Antidepressant Potential of Natural Bioactive Components from Tea," *Food Research International* 158 (August 2022): 111540, https://pubmed.ncbi.nlm.nih.gov /35840236/.

19. A. L. Montejo, et al. "Incidence of sexual dysfunction associated with antidepressant agents: a prospective multicenter study of 1,022 outpatients," *Journal of Clinical Psychiatry* 62 (2001), no. 3 Suppl.: 15.

20. Agnes Higgens et al., "Antidepressant-Associated Sexual Dysfunction: Impact, Effects, and Treatment," *Drug, Healthcare and Patient Safety* 2 (2010): 141–50, https://pubmed.ncbi.nlm.nih.gov/21701626/.

21. A. Smetanka et al., "Pycnogenol Supplementation as an Adjunct Treatment for Antidepressant-Induced Sexual Dysfunction," *Physiology International* 106, no. 1 (March 1, 2019): 59–69, https://pubmed.ncbi.nlm.nih.gov/30888217/.

22. S. Errichi et al., "Supplementation with Pycnogenol® Improves Signs and Symptoms of Menopausal Transition," *Panminerva Medica* 53, no. 3 Suppl. (September 2011): 65–70, https://pubmed.ncbi.nlm.nih.gov/22108479/.

23. V. Darbinyan et al., "Clinical Trial of Rhodiola Rosea L. Extract SHR-5 in the Treatment of Mild to Moderate Depression," *Nordic Journal of Psychiatry* 61, no. 5 (2007): 343–88, https://pubmed.ncbi.nlm.nih.gov/17990195/.

24. Sara Asadi et al., "Beneficial Effects of Nano-Curcumin Supplement on Depression and Anxiety in Diabetic Patients with Peripheral Neuropathy: A Randomized, Double-Blind, Placebo-Controlled Clinical Trial," *Phytotherapy Research* 34, no. 4 (April 2020): 896–903, https://pubmed.ncbi.nlm.nih.gov/31788880/.

25. Buranee Kanchanatawan et al., "Add-on Treatment with Curcumin Has Antidepressive Effects in Thai Patients with Major Depression: Results of a Randomized Double-Blind Placebo-Controlled Study," *Neurotoxicity Research* 33, no. 3 (April 2018): 621–33, https://pubmed.ncbi.nlm.nih.gov/29327213/.

26. Adrian L. Lopresti et al., "Efficacy of Curcumin, and a Saffron/Curcumin Combination for the Treatment of Major Depression: A Randomised, Double-Blind, Placebo-Controlled Study," *Journal of Affective Disorders* 207 (January 1, 2017): 188–96, https://pubmed.ncbi.nlm.nih.gov/27723543/.

27. Jing-Jie Yu et al., "Chronic Supplementation of Curcumin Enhances the Efficacy of Antidepressants in Major Depressive Disorder: A Randomized, Double-Blind,

Placebo-Controlled Pilot Study," *Journal of Clinical Psychopharmacology* 35, no. 4 (August 2015): 406–10, https://pubmed.ncbi.nlm.nih.gov/26066335/.

28. Laura Fusar-Poli et al., "Curcumin for Depression: A Meta-Analysis," *Critical Reviews in Food Science and Nutrition* 60, no. 15 (2020): 2643–53, https://pubmed.ncbi.nlm.nih.gov/31423805/.

29. Qin Xiang Ng et al., "Clinical Use of Curcumin in Depression: A Meta-Analysis," *Journal of American Medical Directors Association* 1, no. 18 (June 1, 2017): 503–08, https://pubmed.ncbi.nlm.nih.gov/28236605/.

CHAPTER 11
Repairing the Gut-Brain Network

1. Karlyle G. Bistas et al., "The Benefits of Prebiotics and Probiotics on Mental Health," *Cureus* 15, no. 8 (August 9, 2023): e43217, https://pubmed.ncbi.nlm.nih.gov/37692658/.

2. Asma Kazemi et al., "Effect of Probiotic and Prebiotic vs Placebo on Psychological Outcomes in Patients with Major Depressive Disorder: A Randomized Clinical Trial," *Clinical Nutrition* 38, no. 2 (April 2019): 522–28, https://pubmed.ncbi.nlm.nih.gov/29731182/.

3. Zeinab Ghorbani et al., "The Effect of Synbiotic as an Adjuvant Therapy to Fluoxetine in Moderate Depression: A Randomized Multicenter Trial," *Archives of Neuroscience* 5, no. 2 (2018): e60507, https://doi.org/10.5812/archneurosci.60507.

4. Maria Ines Pinto-Sanchez et al., "Probiotic Bifidobacterium longum NCC3001 Reduces Depression Scores and Alters Brain Activity: A Pilot Study in Patients with Irritable Bowel Syndrome," *Gastroenterology* 153, no. 2 (August 2017): 448–59.e8, https://pubmed.ncbi.nlm.nih.gov/28483500/.

5. R. F. Slykerman et al., "Effect of Lactobacillus rhamnosus HN001 in Pregnancy on Postpartum Symptoms of Depression and Anxiety: A Randomised Double-Blind Placebo-Controlled Trial," *EbioMedicine* 24 (October 2017): 159–65, https://pubmed.ncbi.nlm.nih.gov/28943228/.

6. José Antonio Pico-Monllor et al., "Influence and Selection of Probiotics on Depressive Disorders in Occupational Health: Scoping Review," *Nutrients* 15, no. 16 (August 11, 2023): 3551, https://pubmed.ncbi.nlm.nih.gov/37630741/.

7. Mariangela Rondanelli et al., "Micronutrients Dietary Supplementation Advices for Celiac Patients on Long-Term Gluten-Free Diet with Good Compliance: A Review," *Medicina* 55, no. 7 (July 3, 2019): 337, https://pubmed.ncbi.nlm.nih.gov/31277328/.

8. Nidhi Sharma et al., "Celiac Disease Poses Significant Risk in Developing Depression, Anxiety, Headache, Epilepsy, Panic Disorder, Dysthymia: A Meta-Analysis," *Indian Journal of Gastroenterology* 40, no. 5 (October 2021): 453–62, https://pubmed.ncbi.nlm.nih.gov/34839445/.

9. Monique Germone et al., "Anxiety and Depression in Pediatric Patients with Ce-

liac Disease: A Large Cross-Sectional Study," *Journal of Pediatric Gastroenterology and Nutrition* 75, no. 2 (August 1, 2022): 181–85, https://pubmed.ncbi.nlm.nih.gov/35641896/.

10. Sara Haj Ali et al., "The Prevalence of Anxiety and Depressive Symptoms Among Patients with Celiac Disease in Jordan," *Cureus* 15, no. 6 (June 1, 2023): e39842, https://pubmed.ncbi.nlm.nih.gov/37397686/ 11.

11. Luchen Shi et al., "Depression and Risk of Infectious Diseases: A Mendelian Randomization Study," *Translational Psychiatry* 14, no. 1 (June 8, 2024): 245, https://pubmed.ncbi.nlm.nih.gov/38851830/.

12. Maja Drewes et al., "Factors Associated with the Diagnosis of Depression in Women Followed in Gynecological Practices in Germany," *Journal of Psychiatric Research* 141 (September 2021): 358–63, https://pubmed.ncbi.nlm.nih.gov/34304041/.

13. Yoon Seol Bae et al., "Short-Term Antifungal Treatments of Caprylic Acid with Carvacrol or Thymol Induce Synergistic 6-Log Reduction of Pathogenic Candida albicans by Cell Membrane Disruption and Efflux Pump Inhibition," *Cellular Physiology and Biochemistry* 53, no. 2 (2019): 285–300, https://pubmed.ncbi.nlm.nih.gov/31334617/.

14. Eric M. Hecht et al., "Cross-Sectional Examination of Ultra-Processed Food Consumption and Adverse Mental Health Symptoms," *Public Health Nutrition* 25, no. 11 (November 2022): 3225–34, https://pubmed.ncbi.nlm.nih.gov/35899785/.

15. Natalia Gomes Goncalves et al., "Association Between Consumption of Ultra-processed Foods and Cognitive Decline," *JAMA Neurology* 80, no. 2 (February 1, 2023): 142–50, https://pubmed.ncbi.nlm.nih.gov/36469335/.

16. Zheyi Song et al., "Effects of Ultra-Processed Foods on the Microbiota-Gut-Brain Axis: The Bread-and-Butter Issue," *Food Research International* 167 (May 2023): 112730, https://pubmed.ncbi.nlm.nih.gov/37087282/.

CHAPTER 12

The Care and Feeding of Your Hormones

1. Sara Odawara et al., "Association of Low-Normal Free T4 Levels with Future Major Depression Development," *Journal of the Endocrine Society* 7, no. 8 (July 20, 2023): bvad096, https://pubmed.ncbi.nlm.nih.gov/37528949/.

2. Laily Najafi et al., "Depressive Symptoms in Patients with Subclinical Hypothyroidism—the Effect of Treatment with Levothyroxine: a Double-Blind Randomized Clinical Trial," *Endocrine Research* 40, no. 3 (2015): 121–26, https://pubmed.ncbi.nlm.nih.gov/25775223/.

3. Jae Hoon Moon et al., "Effect of Increased Levothyroxine Dose on Depressive Mood in Older adults Undergoing Thyroid Hormone Replacement Therapy," *Clinical Endocrinology* 93, no. 2 (August 2020):196–203, https://pubmed.ncbi.nlm.nih.gov/32282957/.

4. Robert Krysiak et al., "Sexual Function and Depressive Symptoms in Young Women with Hypothyroidism Receiving Levothyroxine/Liothyronine Combination Therapy: A Pilot Study," *Current Medical Research and Opinion* 34, no. 9 (September 2018): 1579–86, https://pubmed.ncbi.nlm.nih.gov/29508635/.

5. Shuai Zhao et al., "Increased 10-Year Cardiovascular Disease Risk in Depressed Patients with Coexisting Subclinical Hypothyroidism," *Frontiers in Psychiatry* 14 (July 4, 2023): 1185782, https://pubmed.ncbi.nlm.nih.gov/37469355/.

6. Rakesh Kumar et al., "The Association Between Thyroid Stimulating Hormone and Depression: A Historical Cohort Study," *Mayo Clinic Proceedings* 98, no. 7 (July 2023): 1009–20, https://pubmed.ncbi.nlm.nih.gov/37419569/.

7. Andreas Walther et al., "Association of Testosterone Treatment with Alleviation of Depressive Symptoms in Men: A Systematic Review and Meta-Analysis," *JAMA Psychiatry* 76, no. 1 (January 1, 2019): 31–40, https://pubmed.ncbi.nlm.nih.gov/30427999/.

8. E. Sherwood Brown et al., "A Randomized, Double-Blind, Placebo-Controlled Trial of Pregnenolone for Bipolar Depression," *Neuropsychopharmacology* 39, no. 12 (November 2014): 2867–73, https://pubmed.ncbi.nlm.nih.gov/24917198/.

9. I. Julian Osuji et al., "Pregnenolone for Cognition and Mood in Dual Diagnosis Patients," *Psychiatry Research* 178, no. 2 (July 30, 2010): 309–12, https://pubmed.ncbi.nlm.nih.gov/20493557/.

10. Agorastos Agorastos et al., "Morning Salivary Dehydroepiandrosterone (DHEA) Qualifies as the Only Neuroendocrine Biomarker Separating Depressed Patients with and Without Prior History of Depression: An HPA Axis Challenge Study," *Journal of Psychiatric Research* 161 (May 2023): 449–454, https://pubmed.ncbi.nlm.nih.gov/37059029/.

11. R. J. T. Mocking et al., "DHEAS and Cortisol/DHEAS-Ratio in Recurrent Depression: State, or Trait Predicting 10-Year Recurrence?," *Psychoneuroendocrinology* 59 (September 2015): 91–101, https://pubmed.ncbi.nlm.nih.gov/26036454/.

12. Xiaoling Jiang et al., "Attenuated DHEA and DHEA-S Response to Acute Psychosocial Stress in Individuals with Depressive Disorders," *Journal of Affective Disorders* 215 (June 2017): 118–24, https://pubmed.ncbi.nlm.nih.gov/28319688/.

13. O. M. Wolkowitz et al., "Dehydroepiandrosterone (DHEA) Treatment of Depression," *Biological Psychiatry* 41, no. 3 (February 1, 1997): 311–18, https://pubmed.ncbi.nlm.nih.gov/9024954/.

14. Clayton Peixoto et al., "The Effects of Dehydroepiandrosterone (DHEA) in the Treatment of Depression and Depressive Symptoms in Other Psychiatric and Medical Illnesses: A Systematic Review," *Current Drug Targets* 15, no. 9 (2014): 901–14, https://pubmed.ncbi.nlm.nih.gov/25039497/.

CHAPTER 13
Inner Strengths, Outer Connections

1. Pim Cuijpers et al., "Psychological Treatment of Depression: A Systematic Overview of a 'Meta-Analytic Research Domain,'" *Journal of Affective Disorders* 335 (August 15, 2023): 141–51, https://pubmed.ncbi.nlm.nih.gov/37178828/.

2. Pim Cuijpers et al., "Cognitive Behavior Therapy vs. Control Conditions, Other Psychotherapies, Pharmacotherapies and Combined Treatment for Depression: A Comprehensive Meta-Analysis Including 409 Trials with 52,702 Patients," *World Psychiatry* 22, no. 1 (February 2023): 105–15, https://pubmed.ncbi.nlm.nih.gov /36640411/.

3. Natalie Gukasyan et al., "Efficacy and Safety of Psilocybin-Assisted Treatment for Major Depressive Disorder: Prospective 12-Month Follow-Up," *Journal of Psychopharmacology* 36, no. 2 (February 2022): 151–58, https://pubmed.ncbi.nlm .nih.gov/35166158/.

4. Damian Swieczkowski et al., "Efficacy and Safety of Psilocybin in the Treatment of Major Depressive Disorder (MDD): A Dose-Response Network Meta-Analysis of Randomized Placebo-Controlled Clinical Trials," *Psychiatry Research* 344 (February 2025): 116337, https://pubmed.ncbi.nlm.nih.gov/39754904/.

5. Soroush Oraee et al., "Intranasal Esketamine for Patients with Major Depressive Disorder: A Systematic Review and Meta-Analysis," *Journal of Psychiatric Research* 180 (December 2024): 371–79, https://pubmed.ncbi.nlm.nih.gov/39522447/.

6. Cameron N. Calder et al., "Number Needed to Treat (NNT) for Ketamine and Esketamine in Adults with Treatment-Resistant Depression: A Systematic Review and Meta-Analysis," *Journal of Affective Disorders* 356 (July 1, 2024): 753–62, https://pubmed.ncbi.nlm.nih.gov/38636712/.

7. "Cybin Reports Positive Phase 2 Data for CYB003, Demonstrating Breakthrough 12-Month Efficacy in Treating Major Depressive Disorder," Cybin, November 18, 2024, https://ir.cybin.com/investors/news/news-details/2024/Cybin -Reports-Positive-Phase-2-Data-for-CYB003-Demonstrating-Breakthrough-12 -Month-Efficacy-in-Treating-Major-Depressive-Disorder/default.aspx.

CHAPTER 14
Lifestyle Healing

1. Yujie Zhao et al., "The Brain Structure, Immunometabolic and Genetic Mechanisms Underlying the Association Between Lifestyle and Depression," *Nature Mental Health* 1 (2023): 736–50, https://www.nature.com/articles/s44220-023 -00120-1.

2. M. Walaszek, et al. "Low-carbohydrate diet as a nutritional intervention in major depression disorder: focus on relapse prevention." *Nutritional Neuroscience* 27 (October 2024): 1185–1198.

3. L. Calabrese, at al. "Complete remission of depression and anxiety using a ketogenic diet: case series." *Frontiers in Nutrition* (2024): 11:1396685. Published May 14, 2024.

4. N. Needham, et al. "Pilot study of a ketogenic diet in bipolar disorder," *BJPsych Open* 9 (October 10, 2023): 6.

5. Andreas Heissel et al., "Exercise as Medicine for Depressive Symptoms? A Systematic Review and Meta-Analysis with Meta-Regression," *British Journal of Sports Medicine* 57, no. 16 (August 2023): 1049–57, https://pubmed.ncbi.nlm.nih.gov/36731907/.

6. Matthew Pearce et al., "Association Between Physical Activity and Risk of Depression: A Systematic Review and Meta-Analysis," *JAMA Psychiatry* 79, no. 6 (2022): 550–59, https://pubmed.ncbi.nlm.nih.gov/35416941/.

7. Ulf Ekelund et al., "Does Physical Activity Attenuate, or Even Eliminate, the Detrimental Association of Sitting Time with Mortality? A Harmonised Meta-Analysis of Data from More Than 1 Million Men and Women," *Lancet* 388, no. 10051 (September 24, 2016): 1302–10, https://pubmed.ncbi.nlm.nih.gov/27475271/.

8. Joshua Felton Gilens et al., "Does Light Therapy Decrease Depression in Older Adults?" *American Family Physician*, 104, no. 4 (October 1, 2021): 417–18, https://pubmed.ncbi.nlm.nih.gov/34652110/.

CHAPTER 15

The Integrative Approach to Antidepressants: More Benefit, Less Risk

1. Elham Ranjbar et al., "Effects of Zinc Supplementation on Efficacy of Antidepressant Therapy, Inflammatory Cytokines, and Brain-Derived Neurotrophic Factor in Patients with Major Depression," *Nutritional Neuroscience* 17, no. 2 (February 2014): 65–71, https://pubmed.ncbi.nlm.nih.gov/23602205/.

2. Marcin Siwek et al., "Zinc Supplementation Augments Efficacy of Imipramine in Treatment Resistant Patients: A Double Blind, Placebo-Controlled Study," *Journal of Affective Disorders* 118, no. 1–3 (November 2009): 187–95, https://pubmed.ncbi.nlm.nih.gov/19278731/.

3. Andreas Doing et al., "Zinc as an Adjunct to Antidepressant Medication: A Meta-Analysis with Subgroup Analysis for Different Levels of Treatment Response to Antidepressants," *Nutritional Neuroscience* 25, no. 9 (September 2022): 1785–95, https://pubmed.ncbi.nlm.nih.gov/33641635/.

4. Seema Mehdi et al., "Omega-3 Fatty Acids Supplementation in the Treatment of Depression: An Observational Study," *Journal of Personalized Medicine* 13, no. 2 (January 27, 2023): 224, https://pubmed.ncbi.nlm.nih.gov/36836458/.

5. Kamila Krawczyk et al., "Augmentation of Antidepressants with Unsaturated Fatty Acids Omega-3 in Drug-Resistant Depression," *Psychiatria Polska* 46, no. 4 (July–August 2012): 585–98, https://pubmed.ncbi.nlm.nih.gov/23214161/.

6. Sofia Cussotto et al., "Low Omega-3 Polyunsaturated Fatty Acids Predict Reduced Response to Standard Antidepressants in Patients with Major Depressive Disorder," *Depression and Anxiety* 39, no. 5 (May 2022): 407–18, https://pubmed.ncbi.nlm.nih.gov/35357051/.

7. Leila Jahangard et al., "Influence of Adjuvant Omega-3-Polyunsaturated Fatty Acids on Depression, Sleep, and Emotion Regulation Among Outpatients with Major Depressive Disorders—Results from a Double-Blind, Randomized and Placebo-Controlled Clinical Trial," *Journal of Psychiatric Research* 107 (December 2018): 48–56, https://pubmed.ncbi.nlm.nih.gov/30317101/.

8. Deidre J. Smith et al., "Adjunctive Low-Dose Docosahexaenoic Acid (DHA) for Major Depression: An Open-Label Pilot Trial," *Nutritional Neuroscience* 21, no. 3 (April 2018): 224–28, https://pubmed.ncbi.nlm.nih.gov/28224818/.

9. Reinhilde Zimmer et al., "Effects of 1-Year Treatment with Highly Purified Omega-3 Fatty Acids on Depression After Myocardial Infarction: Results from the OMEGA Trial," *Journal of Clinical Psychiatry* 74, no. 11 (November 2013): e1037–45, https://pubmed.ncbi.nlm.nih.gov/24330904/.

10. Vladimir Maletic et al., "A Review of l-Methylfolate as Adjunctive Therapy in the Treatment of Major Depressive Disorder," *Primary Care Companion for CNS Disorders* 25, no. 3 (May 9, 2023): 22nr03361, https://pubmed.ncbi.nlm.nih.gov/37192264/.

11. Wenming Zhao et al., "The Protective Effect of Vitamin D Supplementation as Adjunctive Therapy to Antidepressants on Brain Structural and Functional Connectivity of Patients with Major Depressive Disorder: A Randomized Controlled Trial," *Psychological Medicine* 54, no. 10 (July 2024): 2403–13, https://pubmed.ncbi.nlm.nih.gov/38482853/.

12. John M. Zajecka et al., "Long-Term Efficacy, Safety, and Tolerability of L-Methylfolate Calcium 15 mg as Adjunctive Therapy with Selective Serotonin Reuptake Inhibitors: A 12-Month, Open-Label Study Following a Placebo-Controlled Acute Study," *Journal of Clinical Psychiatry* 77, no. 5 (May 2016): 654–60, https://pubmed.ncbi.nlm.nih.gov/27035404/.

13. George I. Papakostas et al., "Effect of Adjunctive L-Methylfolate 15 mg Among Inadequate Responders to SSRIs in Depressed Patients Who Were Stratified by Biomarker Levels and Genotype: Results from a Randomized Clinical Trial," *Journal of Clinical Psychiatry* 75, no. 8 (August 2014): 855–63, https://pubmed.ncbi.nlm.nih.gov/24813065/.

14. Masoumeh Nazarinasab et al., "Investigating the Effect of Magnesium Supplement in Patients with Major Depressive Disorder Under Selective Serotonin Reuptake Inhibitor Treatment," *Journal of Family Medicine and Primary Care* 11, no. 12 (December 2022): 7800–05, https://pubmed.ncbi.nlm.nih.gov/36994048/.

15. Michał Skalski et al., "Pharmaco-Electroencephalography-Based Assessment of Antidepressant Drug Efficacy—The Use of Magnesium Ions in the Treatment of Depression," *Journal of Clinical Medicine* 10, no. 14 (July 15, 2021): 3135, https://pubmed.ncbi.nlm.nih.gov/34300299/.

16. Beata Ryszewska-Pokrasniewicz et al., "Effects of Magnesium Supplementation on Unipolar Depression: A Placebo-Controlled Study and Review of the Importance of Dosing and Magnesium Status in the Therapeutic Response," *Nutrients* 10, no. 8 (August 3, 2018): 1014, https://pubmed.ncbi.nlm.nih.gov/30081500/.

17. J. Craig Nelson et al., "A Systematic Review and Meta-Analysis of Lithium Augmentation of Tricyclic and Second Generation Antidepressants in Major Depression," *Journal of Affective Disorders* 168 (October 2014): 269–75, https://pubmed.ncbi.nlm.nih.gov/25069082/.

18. Viktoriya Nikolova et al., "Acceptability, Tolerability, and Estimates of Putative Treatment Effects of Probiotics as Adjunctive Treatment in Patients with Depression: A Randomized Clinical Trial," *JAMA Psychiatry* 80, no. 8 (August 1, 2023): 842–47, https://pubmed.ncbi.nlm.nih.gov/37314797/.

19. Viktoriya Nikolova et al., "Updated Review and Meta-Analysis of Probiotics for the Treatment of Clinical Depression: Adjunctive vs. Stand-Alone Treatment," *Journal of Clinical Medicine* 10, no. 4 (February 8, 2021): 647, https://pubmed.ncbi.nlm.nih.gov/33567631/.

20. Lili Gao et al., "Antidepressants Effects of Rhodiola Capsule Combined with Sertraline for Major Depressive Disorder: A Randomized Double-Blind Placebo-Controlled Clinical Trial," *Journal of Affective Disorders* 265 (March 15, 2020): 99–103, https://pubmed.ncbi.nlm.nih.gov/32090788/.

21. W. O. Monteiro, et al. "Anorgasmia from clomipramine in obsessive–compulsive disorder: a controlled trial," *The British Journal of Psychiatry* 151 (1; 1987): 107–112.

22. Agnes Higgens et al., "Antidepressant-Associated Sexual Dysfunction: Impact, Effects, and Treatment," *Drug, Healthcare and Patient Safety* 2 (September 9, 2010): 141–50, https://pubmed.ncbi.nlm.nih.gov/21701626/.

23. Smetanka et al., "Pycnogenol Supplementation as an Adjunct Treatment for Antidepressant-Induced Sexual Dysfunction."

24. Yu et al., "Chronic Supplementation of Curcumin Enhances the Efficacy of Antidepressants in Major Depressive Disorder."

CHAPTER 16

Understanding Antidepressant Deprescribing

1. Rachel Aviv, "The Challenge of Going Off Psychiatric Drugs," *The New Yorker*, April 1, 2019, https://www.newyorker.com/magazine/2019/04/08/the-challenge-of-going-off-psychiatric-drugs.

2. Lawrence E. K. Altman, "Valium, Most Prescribed Drug, Is Center of a Medical Dispute," *The New York Times*, May 19, 1974, https://www.nytimes.com/1974/05/19/archives/valium-most-prescribed-drug-is-center-of-a-medical-dispute-wide-use.html.

3. Medicines and Healthcare Products Regulatory Agency, summary of the meeting of the Committee on Safety of Medicines, held on Thursday, March 26, 1998,

London, U.K., http://www.mhra.gov.uk/home/groups/l-cs-el/documents/committeedocument/con003341.pdf.

4. Medicines and Healthcare Products Regulatory Agency, minutes of the meeting of the CSM Expert Group on the Safety of SRRIs, held on Tuesday, July 22, 2003, London, U.K.

5. Giovanni A. Fava et al., "Withdrawal Symptoms After Selective Serotonin Reuptake Inhibitor Discontinuation: A Systematic Review," *Psychotherapy and Psychosomatics* 84, no. 2 (2015): 72–81, https://pubmed.ncbi.nlm.nih.gov/25721705/.

6. John Read, "Withdrawal from Antidepressants: A Review," *Psychology Today*, October 26, 2020, https://www.psychologytoday.com/us/blog/psychiatry-through-the-looking-glass/202010/withdrawal-antidepressants-review.

7. Manish K. Jha et al., "When Discontinuing SSRI Antidepressants Is a Challenge: Management Tips," *American Journal of Psychiatry* 175, no. 12 (December 1, 2018): 1176–84, https://pubmed.ncbi.nlm.nih.gov/30501420/.

8. Jim van Os et al., "Outcomes of Hyperbolic Tapering of Antidepressants," *Therapeutic Advances in Psychopharmacology* 13 (May 9, 2023): 20451253231171518, https://pubmed.ncbi.nlm.nih.gov/37200818/.

9. Mark Abie Horowitz et al., "Case-Based Learning: Safe Withdrawal and Tapering of Antidepressants," *The Pharmaceutical Journal*, September 19, 2023, https://pharmaceutical-journal.com/article/ld/case-based-learning-safe-withdrawal-and-tapering-of-antidepressants.

INDEX

ABOUT THE AUTHORS

A pioneer in the field of functional medicine, **JAMES M. GREENBLATT, MD,** has treated patients since 1988. He is the founder of Psychiatry Redefined, and is an assistant clinical professor of psychiatry at Tufts University School of Medicine and Dartmouth College Geisel School of Medicine. Dr. Greenblatt has lectured internationally on the scientific evidence for nutritional interventions in psychiatry and mental illness and is a leading contributor to helping physicians and patients understand the role of personalized medicine for mental illness. He is the author of eight books, including *Finally Focused: The Breakthrough Natural Treatment Plan for ADHD.*

BILL GOTTLIEB, CPHC, is one of America's most successful health book authors and journalists, a certified professional health coach, and a media personality. He has authored and coauthored sixteen published books, which have sold over three million copies and been translated into eleven languages.